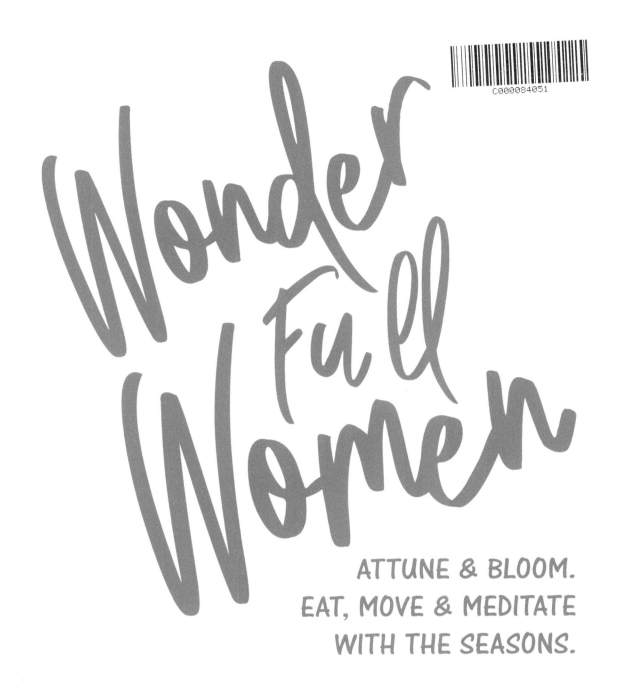

Wonder Full Women

ATTUNE & BLOOM.
EAT, MOVE & MEDITATE
WITH THE SEASONS.

FREYA BENNETT-OVERSTALL

Balboa Press books may be ordered through booksellers or by contacting:

Balboa Press
A Division of Hay House
1663 Liberty Drive
Bloomington, IN 47403
www.balboapress.com.au
AU TFN: 1 800 844 925 (Toll Free inside Australia)
AU Local: 0283 107 086 (+61 2 8310 7086 from outside Australia)

Interior Image Credit: Shutterstock, Ali Mayfield & Freya Bennett-Overstall

ISBN: 978-1-9822-9382-6 (sc)
ISBN: 978-1-9822-9383-3 (e)

Print information available on the last page.

Balboa Press rev. date: 05/31/2022

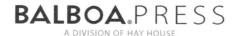

BALBOA.PRESS
A DIVISION OF HAY HOUSE

Humbly and lovingly, to Caroline.

Contents

Foreword

Thirty years ago, Freya and I were incidentally but fortuitously paired, in what was my third and her first year of chiropractic study. We shared notes and stories. She appreciated my insights from being already a few years into the course, but how beneficial for me to be partnered with someone from such a contrasting background to my own. Years before she would write this book, she was already opening my mind in subtle ways. Freya's life experiences had been such that she thought it not unusual to have always been versed in the world of meditation, yoga, and Buddhist practices. I believe travelling, frequently changing schools and locations, have taught her the necessity and benefit of continual adaptation. I feel it gave her an openness to her surrounding environment and people, even as they constantly changed. She lived a life attuned to the seasons and her environment even before she was aware of it.

Over these years of friendship, I have seen the evolution of Freya. She's never been one to pass up an adventure. She's delved into the study of different techniques to enhance her innate healing abilities, and she's thrived in the adaptation of her skills to wherever life has taken her. I've had the pleasure of treating mutual patients and can attest to their loyal gratitude for her incredible chiropractic skills in healing both mind and body. I was not alone in experiencing immense sadness that her chiropractic years might not continue after her autoimmune diagnosis. To see Freya not be able to impart her healing gifts to others felt such a tremendous loss. But on the contrary, her skills just evolved to an even more complex level. The way in which she has incorporated so uniquely all these attributes is something you are about to be gifted with in reading this book.

Freya has collated all the wisdom absorbed from her upbringing with the study of health science, philosophy, and the body's innate ability to heal itself. She's gained further knowledge and skills in complementary areas, like meditation, mindfulness, yoga, and traditional Chinese medicine. She's studied other cultures to find the collective knowledge long known individually but not necessarily assembled around the rhythm of our seasons. Her curiosity and observation of nature and its inhabitants will be thought-provoking for you. You will find the personal expression of this understanding and her insights, combined with science, in *Wonder Full Women*.

This book will help you listen to and understand yourself, by learning how to engage with the rhythm of your body in its present environment as you flow from one season to the next. It is a practical guide that you can refer to time and time again. The meditation and yoga sequences are carefully constructed so that you can flourish and, as Freya so aptly says, attune and bloom. I'm proud to have the opportunity to recommend it to you.

Dr Tania Kennelly
Chiropractor

Introduction

The seed of this book was first planted by a dear friend of mine who asked me, "What three things have helped you [heal] most?

I haven't been able to distil it down to three things. But following her question, along with queries from friends, patients, and students, a book has sprouted and grown.

Within these pages, I offer ancient wisdom practices and suggestions to help us eat, move, and meditate with the seasons. They allow us to attune to the inevitable changes of our natural surroundings, life's challenges, and ourselves. They help us cultivate calm, connection, wonder, and well-being.

As the title suggests, this book has been written with women in mind. However, it is for everyone, and I hope that all gender and ages find some help and/or interesting ideas within.

This book is by no means exhaustive. I continue to learn, grow, and heal each day. Please remember we are all different and it's important to bring a gentle curiosity to each offering. What might help you today might not help tomorrow and vice versa. I encourage you to tune in daily, both to yourself and your surrounding environment. I wish you all the best with your practice.

Attune and bloom.

How to Best Use This Book

I suggest you start by reading this book cover to cover. There are *essential topics* covered in the early chapters, in Part I, that are the building blocks of the *seasonal practices* found in Part II. You can then easily choose to return to specific sections as needed. Each seasonal chapter contains inspirational words, beneficial movement, meditation, and seasonal food and preparation.

This symbol is to let you know there is an audible recording available. I have recorded various guided meditations, and you can access them for free via Insight Timer – https://insighttimer.com/freya

This symbol is to let you know there is a video recording of the practice available. You can find these videos on my website – https://www.freyabennettoverstall.com/

Commonly used abbreviations and Sanskrit translations can be found at the end of the book.

My Personal Journey

I was born in lush tropical North Queensland, Tjapukai (Djabugay) Country. I spent many happy hours outside in my natural environment playing, exploring, and imagining. My dad and stepmum grew most of the vegetables we ate, along with delicious fruit from tropical trees.

I was blessed to be introduced to yoga, tai chi, and dance at an early age, and they became regular mindful movement styles I used in my life. I was about five years old when my mum was first introduced to Tibetan Buddhism, and so I started accompanying her to Tara House and later to Chenrezig Institute. A few years later, I went off on my first weekend yoga retreat.

When I was a young girl, my mum and I often moved between Far North Queensland and Melbourne—the top tropical corner of the Eastern coast to the bottom temperate oceanic corner. My main years of high school were spent in Brisbane, Southern Queensland.

Eventually, university took me back down to Melbourne. There, I spent five years studying and another year practising chiropractic in sleepy beachside Mount Martha. During my first year of university, a girlfriend introduced me to African dance. I was later honoured to be invited to join and perform with Mzuri Dancers, led and choreographed by Suzanne Mzuri Watts. Oh, how the drums and the movement style made my body and heart sing!

These six years in Melbourne—full of dance, yoga, a two-month stint in India, the early death of three friends, university study, and chiropractic practice—all explored and further highlighted the miracle of the human body to me. I learned about innate intelligence and the importance of taking good care of one's body and appreciating this one precious life.

In 1999, Europe was calling, and I headed off to my dad's country of birth, England. I spent many happy, sweaty hours African dancing in London, Paris and, later, under a mango tree in Abene, the Casamance region of Senegal. This was alongside practising as a chiropractor in central London. I began to teach mindfulness of breath practices to my patients, to help them with sleep and stress reduction. I also fell deeply in love with an Englishman, who is now my husband. I was filling my cup with dance, meditation, yoga, travel, love, and helping others.

In 2004, we waved a teary goodbye to London and travelled overland through wild and wonder full Africa. We spent three marvellous months out of our comfort zone, awestruck by the animals, the natural surrounding beauty, and the harshness of existence experienced by most. We arrived in Melbourne in early 2005 and were soon blessed with two scrumptious boys born a couple of years apart.

In 2013, I had a drastically empty cup. I found myself stuck in the depleting habit of wanting to please and help everyone but myself. I had young boys, I was working part-time as a chiropractor, and I was volunteering at the school. We were selling one home and buying another. I was grieving the death of my father while also being the executor of his will, my sister in-law was diagnosed with breast cancer, and my husband was working superlong hours as a surgeon (so it often felt like I was solo parenting). Phew! It makes me feel exhausted just writing this.

My own self-care became a past memory, and I was definitely not included on my "to-do list." I was terrible at asking for and accepting help—until my body screamed at me to stop. And it truly stopped me. It physically stopped me. I lost strength and full use of my right arm. I could no longer carry our youngest son. Even giving a hug was physically painful and difficult. I couldn't sleep. A neurosurgeon diagnosed two cervical disc protrusions and advised me to stop working immediately. I had never realised how attached I was to my title of *chiropractor* until then.

A roller coaster of a year followed, involving a walking stick, numerous investigative tests, and six months as an outpatient at Cabrini Hospital to retrain my left leg and both arms. Eventually it concluded with a diagnosis of multiple sclerosis (MS).

It was a tough time for my family, and I had a tough lesson to learn—how to fit my own oxygen mask first. I had to learn how to ask for help and graciously accept it. I learnt slowly. Importantly, I also began to remember how to refill my cup and make my heart sing. I started meditating again, painting, and reading anything positive related to recovery from MS. I modified my diet. I found a supportive group of various health practitioners and Tara House Healing Group.

I found my daily formal meditation practice, retreats, yin yoga, and inversions so helpful that I went on to train as a meditation and yoga teacher. I specialised in working with women and children as a chiropractor, so it felt natural to extend this to my meditation and yoga teaching. I started teaching mindful movement and meditation to primary school children in 2015 and began offering classes to women in 2017.

My story is, unfortunately, not uncommon. There are many people suffering from "empty cups" in our fast-paced society. *Wonder Full Women* shares ways I've found to reconnect and to heal my body, heart, and mind and, in doing so, fill my cup. I sincerely hope and wish that this book helps many other women to do so too.

Part I

Ancient Wisdom and the Seasons

Chapter 1
Ancient Wisdom

We belong to the ground
It is our power and we must stay
Close to it or maybe
We will get lost."
—Narritjin Maymuru, born in Arnhem Land, Northern Territory[1]

Our precious planet has many ancient cultures that still exist today. I've found that many of these cultures contain ancient threads that all tie together. Despite their differences in geography and time, they all come to similar understandings and conclusions. They all cultivate an understanding and respect for their natural surrounding environment and its seasons. This has allowed them to adapt, survive, and thrive.

In this book I share some of the timeworn knowledge and practices from ancient Indigenous Australian, Chinese, Indian, and Tibetan cultures.

Indigenous Australian records are continually being discovered and backdated; their culture is now recognised as the oldest living civilisation on our planet. The more recent archaeological finds have discovered this culture has existed for at least sixty-five thousand years. So Australian Aboriginal people have been listening to Country for an awe-inspiringly long time. Country is more than the land and the earth to Australian Aboriginal people. It is a term used to describe both a place of belonging and a way of believing. It embraces all living things, the seasons, stories and great spirit ancestors.

Yoga originated in ancient India. There is no consensus on the exact chronology of yoga. Some suggest it originated in the Indus Valley (3300–1900 BCE) or during the Vedic periods (1500–500 BCE). Regardless of its exact start time, we know yoga to be ancient! The word *yoga* comes from Sanskrit, and it translates as "to yoke," "to join," or "to unite." Many people think of yoga as just the poses—the *asanas*—but this is only one limb of yoga. Yoga has eight limbs. The other seven limbs are *yamas* (five moral restraints), *niyamas* (five observances), *pranayama* (mindful breathing), *pratyahara* (turning inward), *dharana* (concentration, cultivation of attention), *dhyana* (meditation) and *samadhi* (union, absolute oneness).

Buddhism also originated in India, in 500 BC. It spread throughout much of Asia and is now known and practised worldwide. It is based on the original teachings attributed to Gautama Buddha.

Taoism is a philosophical and spiritual tradition that originated in China. Its roots go back to at least 400 BCE. Ancient sages of China first started recording the principles of *Tao* about five thousand years ago.

From the second through to the eighteenth century, travel and trade occurred along the Silk Road. This road connected the East and West. The result of this connection can be seen in similarities between different Asian medicines and practices.

An important key to health and longevity, as acknowledged and respected by these ancient cultures, is to live in harmony with our local community and its surrounding environment. I feel it is important for us to return to and learn from these surviving cultures.

Interconnection

Many of us currently live in cities, and it's easy to become disconnected from the land and its seasons. We have temperature-controlled rooms and cars, electricity allowing light at all hours, and screens constantly glowing and pinging to get our attention. Despite the many gadgets and apps available to quickly connect us, we are, ironically, often left feeling disconnected and alone. We have forgotten the importance of our natural environment and community. Thankfully, there is change afoot and strong stirrings of desire to reconnect.

Interconnection is a recurring theme in many ancient cultures. We are not separate or inconsequential. We are part of something big. If we grasp this and tune in to our environment and ourselves, then we thrive and bloom. Knowing that we are part of everything means we care, and compassion grows for all.

Ancient Australian Aboriginal history and belief has been passed on through songs, poetry, storytelling, and yarning. Yarning involves having a conversation and listening within a group. It involves passing on cultural knowledge and building respectful relationships. They believe that all life—human, animal, bird, and fish—is part of one vast network of relationships, which can be traced to the great spirit ancestors. The spirit ancestors are believed to govern the seasons and, therefore, the growth of natural vegetation, the natural reproduction of animal species, and the cycle of life from birth to death. "Everything in creation is sentient and carries knowledge, therefore everything is deserving of our respect" (shared by Tyson Yunkaporta).[2]

Similarly in Buddhism, connection is often taught through the teaching *pratityasamutpada*, a Sanskrit word that translates as "dependent arising" or "interdependent arising." The basic principle is that all things arise or exist in dependence upon other things, causes, and conditions. Nothing exists in and of itself. This applies to mental and psychological factors, as well as to tangible and intangible things. We are all connected to and interdependent on each other and our environment.

As taught by His Holiness the Fourteenth Dalai Lama (HHDL), at first glance, things may look independent. But when you look deeper, you see that nothing is as it first appears. We are all made up of the same teeny tiny energy particles. In 2015, HHDL came together with a group of quantum physicists and scientists to further discuss and find any commonalities.

Quantum physics, first developed in the twentieth century, seeks to define and understand that which we cannot see or measure. It is the study of the behaviour of matter and energy made up at the molecular, atomic, nuclear, and even smaller microscopic levels. Quantum physics demonstrates that energy is beyond everything that is tangible and material. The idea that we are made up of energy is one of the pillars of connection between quantum physics and spirituality.

Revered Vietnamese Buddhist monk Thich Nhat Hanh provides an example full of wonder at our interconnection in his book *Teachings on Love*: "When we look deeply into a flower, we can see the sun, the clouds, seeds, the nutrients in the soil, and many other things. We understand that the flower cannot exist as a separate, independent self. It is made entirely of what we can call 'non-flower elements' … I am made of non-me elements … Nothing can exist by itself alone. Everything has to inter-be with everything else in the cosmos."[3]

When I share the basic idea or concept of interconnection with primary school children, I invite each student to take a piece of fruit or a snack out of their lunch box and bring it with them as we all join together in a circle. Before we go ahead and eat, I ask the children, one by one, to describe what food they have, where they think it came from, and what was involved with its production, along with how many people they think may have been involved in getting this item of food into their lunch box. It doesn't take long before "light bulbs" go off and small eyes are widening at the realisation of just how interdependent we all are. This segues beautifully into the practice of gratitude (which we will explore further in chapter 4).

Basics of Taoism

There was something formless yet complete
That existed before heaven and earth;
Without a sound, without substance,
Dependent on nothing, unchanging,
All-pervading, unfailing.
One may think of it as the mother
Of all things under heaven.
It's true name I do not know;
"Tao" is the nickname I give it.

—Lao Tzu

These mysterious words are from the poem *Tao Te Ching* written in China almost 2,500 years ago by the poet and philosopher Lao Tzu.[4] He is believed to be the founder of Taoism.

Tao (pronounced /dao/dow/) translates as the "Way." As described by Daniel Reid in his book *The Tao of Health, Sex, and Longevity*, "Tao is the universal and enduring Way of Nature."[5]

Ancient Chinese sages studied the relationships and patterns of nature closely. They then applied these universal findings to the human ecosystem. They recognised the human body as a microcosm of the universe. This close observation of the patterns of nature and reality led to the formation of the five element theory.

By living in harmony with the "Way," a person will not have to fight against the universe's natural flow. It is believed that, by learning to harmonise with the Tao, you may harness its power to enhance and prolong your life. If you live in harmony with the Way, you will benefit, whereas, if you struggle against the Way (things are) you will suffer.

To quote Daniel Reid again, "To go against Tao is like trying to swim upstream against a strong current—sooner or later you will exhaust your energy, grind to a halt and be swept away by the cosmic currents of Tao."[6]

The primary characteristic of the Way is constant change. Taoism sees the universe in a state of constant flux. Everything is interrelated, interactive, and interdependent for existence. The interaction of yin and yang, the union of opposites, is Tao.

Yin and Yang

Yin Yang Symbol

The Taoists observed that everything has yin or yang attributes. Yin and yang are relative terms. There is no absolute yin and no absolute yang. They complement each other and cannot exist without each other. Each comes from the other and includes part of the other. Can you notice the seed of each in the above symbol? Everything contains the seed of its opposite.

For example, the crest of a wave is yang, and its trough is yin. The sunny side of a mountain is yang; the shadowed side is yin. Yin is the darker side of things. Yang is the lighter side of things. We can't see the light without the dark. We need both to be able to find balance.

It is important to remember that yin and yang are relative. If we have an ice-cold glass of water next to a room temperature glass of water, the ice-cold water will be yin, and the room temperature water will be yang; *but* if we have a hot glass of water next to a room temperature glass of water, then the room temperature glass is yin and the hot water is yang.

Foods have both yin and yang properties, as does the body and our natural environment. Cool autumn and cold winter are yin, warm spring and hot summer are yang. Movement can also be described as yin and yang.

Table 1.1 Yin and Yang

Yin	Yang
Dark	Light
Cold	Hot
Moon	Sun
Damp	Dry
Deficient	Excessive
Deep	Superficial
Passive	Active
Female	Male
Lower	Upper
Solid/Full	Hollow/Empty
Inside	Outside

Domination of either yin or yang results in imbalance. Our modern world is very yang, very active. It rarely reflects balance. We tend to go, go, go. We have been conditioned into thinking that being busy is a sign of success. Constant marketing campaigns and social media often leave us wanting and feeling like we are not enough.

As cancer, heart disease, autoimmune disease, and mental illness rates rise rapidly, more people are looking for preventive and holistic measures. More people are looking for ways to cultivate a balanced lifestyle; this often involves inviting more yin into their life.

I am lucky enough to call Paul Bedson one of my teachers, from my time studying at the Yarra Valley Living Centre. He writes so eloquently and has graciously allowed me to share this with you: "It is so important to allow ourselves some time and space to listen to the still, quiet voice inside. To slow down, to tune in to the *yin* in a busy *yang* world. This is the voice of our inner integrity, our inner knowing and discrimination. We all share this voice, it is the voice of our common humanity and our shared spirit."

Finding a balance between both is the key. We can only be yang-like for so long before crashing, and we can only be yin-like for so long before stagnating.

Chi

The ancient Chinese described *chi* (pronounced /chee/) as the vital essence found in all things, in both matter and energy. *Chi* is similar to the term *prana* (life force) from India, *lung* from Tibet, and also *ki* from Japan.

Chi is an invisible force that constantly meanders through our bodies and our environment. It is a concept that helps to describe every aspect of life. It is thought to be what causes our hearts to beat, our brains to think, plants to grow, and planets to rotate.

In relation to food, if it is of good quality chi, the food is fresh, will taste better, and will be most nourishing. In relation to the body, good quality chi manifests as a lack of obstruction in the body, which results in better functioning of organs, circulation, emotions, and mind. Any stimulus—such as exercise/movement; bodywork (adjustment, manipulation, acupuncture, neuroemotional technique (NET), cupping, applied kinesiology (AK), Rolfing, massage, and so on); herbal therapy; food; pranayama; and meditation—that releases or balances the flow of chi will result in healing.

"If it is not moving, it is not healing." This from Jo Phee, another of my revered teachers, the founder and main teacher of Yinspiration.[7]

Meridians

Meridians (or *nadis* from India, *sen* lines from Thailand) are the channels along which chi flows in the body. They create a network throughout the body. If this network is blocked or disrupted, the body will not function properly. This network can be thought of as a map that shows the subtle energies that flow within us.

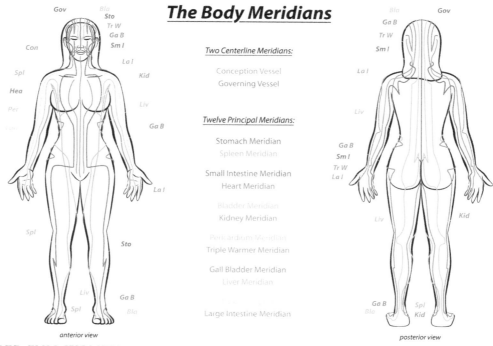

The Body Meridians

Two Centerline Meridians:

Conception Vessel
Governing Vessel

Twelve Principal Meridians:

Stomach Meridian
Spleen Meridian
Small Intestine Meridian
Heart Meridian
Bladder Meridian
Kidney Meridian
Pericardium Meridian
Triple Warmer Meridian
Gall Bladder Meridian
Liver Meridian
Large Intestine Meridian

anterior view

posterior view

Within TCM (traditional Chinese medicine), there are seventy-one meridians; fourteen are considered most important. We will explore the twelve principal meridians in this book (known as *Jing Mai*). There are six meridians that begin or end in the feet, the lower body. And there are six meridians that begin or end in the hands, the upper body. Each yin meridian (storage organ) is paired up with a yang meridian (hollow organ).

Healthy chi flows in certain directions through these twelve meridians. Chi enters the meridian system at the Lung meridians and flows from one meridian to the next, taking a full twenty-four hours to complete one cycle throughout the body. Meridian tapping, a process of tapping the body in the direction of healthy chi flow along the chosen meridian, is introduced later in this book.

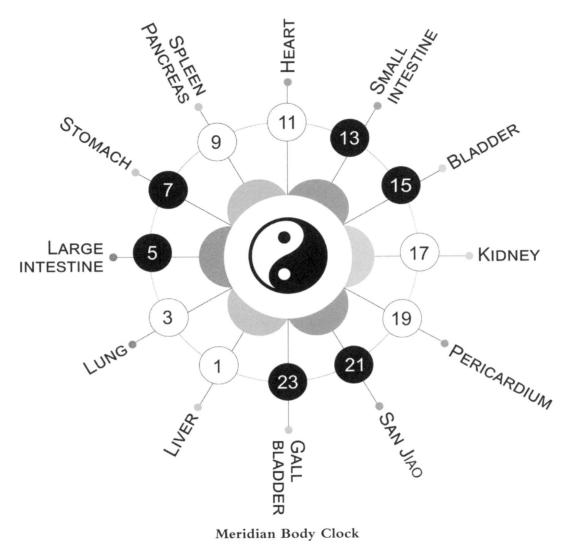

Meridian Body Clock

It is important to know that the Taoist concept of organs is not the same as in Western medicine. For example, a western kidney is not a Chinese Kidney. Western medicine offers a more reductive view, looking at the specific anatomical structure of the organ. In TCM, the physical organ plus its systemic tissue, different energetic qualities, and psycho-emotional components are all considered. When you see the word *Kidney* in this book with a capital "K," it refers to the Chinese organ concept and meridians, which deals with the function and network of the Kidney, including the adrenal glands, rather than the physical kidney organ as we know it in the West.

Table 1.2. Chinese Organ Systems Table

Meridian	Body Position	Function	Emotion
Lung (yin)	Upper/arm	Immunity, respiration (expiration), regulation of the balance of moisture in the body	Sadness, grief
Large Intestine (yang)	Upper/arm	Involved with transportation, transformation, and elimination	Dogmatic, feeling stuck
Stomach (yang)	Lower/leg	Reservoir for food and water, digestion, descending energy	Over-sympathetic, nervous
Spleen (includes pancreas) (yin)	Lower/leg	Metabolism, nourishment, lifting energy	Low self-esteem, worry
Heart (yin)	Upper/arm	Circulation, nervous system, consciousness/Shen	Frightfully overjoyed, manic, anxious
Small Intestine (yang)	Upper/arm	Receives and stores food and water	Lost, vulnerable
Urinary Bladder (yang)	Lower/leg	Stores and discharges urine	Paralysed will, feelings of inefficiency
Kidney (includes adrenals) (yin)	Lower/leg	Water metabolism, stores Jing, longevity, physical and mental maturation, reproduction, bone health	Fear, dread
Pericardium (yin)	Upper/arm	Circulation, protects the heart, guides hormones and sexual functions	Difficulty expressing and feeling emotions, depression
Triple Warmer (does not involve a physical organ; it is a collection of body functions) (yang)	Upper/arm	Controls internal heat and maintains organ functions	Overwhelm
Gall Bladder (yang)	Lower/leg	Reservoir for bile	Resentment, feeling galled
Liver (yin)	Lower/leg	Detoxification, blood storage and circulation, emotional regulation, flexibility	Anger, frustration

Five Element Theory

Wuxing is widely translated as "five phases" or "five elements". Each of the twelve principal meridians described above correspond to one of the five elements of TCM. The five element theory is a massive and complicated area of study. I remember feeling completely overwhelmed by its enormity when I first learned about it. (I was in my fifth year at university studying chiropractic and the technique of applied kinesiology.) So here I will offer a brief introduction and explanation. I hope I offer enough information for you to understand its value and, perhaps, spark your interest to investigate further.

The traditional Western definition holds that elements are inert objects. In TCM the five elements are active forces that interplay with each other. The five element theory serves as an aid for understanding life's limitless connections. It shows the interrelationship between the human body and the natural environment. The relationship of each of the elements is key to our health. Each element is intrinsically connected to internal organs, emotions, body parts, and the environment.

Table 1.3. Five Element Table

Element	Wood	Fire	Earth	Metal	Water
Season	Spring	Summer	Late summer	Autumn	Winter
Yin organ	Liver	Heart	Spleen	Lung	Kidney
Yang organ	Gall bladder	Small intestine	Stomach	Large intestine	Urinary bladder

This table shows the five elements matched up with the five yin organs (solid) and their yang (hollow) partners. Each element is also linked to a season. During each season the corresponding organs are considered more vulnerable, so it is beneficial to take measures to nourish them. We can nourish ourselves during each season with particular food, movement, and meditation. (These will be explored in greater detail in the following specific season chapters in Part II.)

Each of the five elements are in a constant state of flux and change. They cannot exist without each other, and they influence each other. There are two healthy cycles; creation and control, and two unhealthy cycles; destruction and insult. The unhealthy cycles occur when creation or control become excessive.

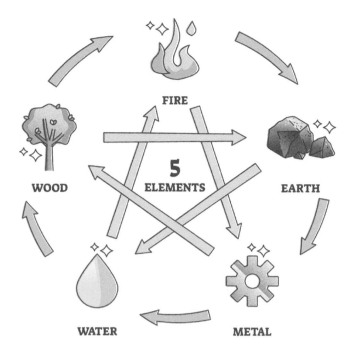

Cycles and Interactions of the Five Elements

Each element is generated by another as shown in the creation cycle, just like a mother supporting and feeding a child. For example, wood burns to generate fire. Fire produces ash, which generates earth.

The control cycle, also known as the father cycle, shows how each element is suppressed or controlled by another. For example, water suppresses fire by extinguishing it. Fire controls metal by melting it.

An example of a destruction cycle, excess father, is when stress-filled, fear-ridden Kidneys (of the water element) fail to remove excess water in the body, which then extinguishes the Heart spirit (of the fire element) and its normal expressions of love and joy. By restoring and balancing Kidney chi, tremendous joy and elation is often felt, and dark clouds of fear are lifted.

Chapter 2
The Seasons

The seasons have a profound cyclical effect on human growth and well-being. We are part of the patterns, cycles, and seasons we see around us. Scientific research is catching up to what has been observed and felt for thousands of years—our physiology is impacted by our surrounding environment.

As ancient wisdom reminds us, everything in nature is connected and in a continuous state of change. Change is the one constant we can be certain of in our life, as much as we may dislike it. When we consciously prepare for and observe the change brought on by each season, we can transform the change into a time of beauty and comfort, even during winter.

Regularly exploring and paying attention to the cycles and seasons of our natural environment can allow us to see that life's beauty is inseparable from its fragility. Important lessons can be learned. We can awaken and connect to being part of something bigger than just oneself. We are not alone, we *all* experience cycles, growth, suffering, joy, and the different seasons of life. There is a season to be born, a season to grow and transform, a season of harvest and storage (of knowledge and wisdom), and eventually there is a season to die.

"Nature isn't something you visit on the weekends—it's what we are deeply part of all the time" (author unknown).

As a young girl, I grew up being distinctly aware of two main seasons—wet and dry. I grew up in tropical north Queensland, Australia.

I have memories of feeling like I was soggily moving through warm soup during the wet season. We had no air conditioning back then. All movement during the wet season felt like it was in "slow mode." Each dusk erupted in a cacophony of song from frogs, insects, and cicadas. As the sun went down, the mosquitoes came out to feed.

The influence of water was on strong display during the wet season. The Barron Falls (aboriginal: *Din Din*) would transform from the dry season's trickle to the wet season's rushing torrent of power, cascading over rocky cliffs. We also had to be careful of cyclones during this time. Throughout my childhood I experienced a few episodes of tying down roofs and stocking up on tinned food, batteries, and other provisions in preparation for a cyclone. It was hot and damp. The wind felt wicked. And we were mere mortals.

I noticed that the dry season allowed for more human energy expenditure. It allowed everyone to dry out and become more productive. The mornings and evenings were cool; we were all less "sticky." Our surrounding natural environment was less forceful during the dry season.

As an adult I have spent most of my time living in Melbourne, Australia, or England. It was here that I first became aware of the presence of five seasons. This book shares and explores the seasons of spring, summer, late summer, autumn and winter, as described in five element theory in TCM.

Table 2.1. Five Element Seasons

	Spring	Summer	Late summer	Autumn	Winter
Element	Wood	Fire	Earth	Metal	Water
Development	Birth	Growth	Transformation	Harvest	Store
Environmental influence	Wind	Heat	Damp	Dry	Cold
Colour	Green	Red	Yellow	White	Black / Dark Blue

Seasonal and Lifestyle Impact on Our Bodies

Our body responds to where we live geographically and to our local seasons. Findings published in an article in *Nature Communications* show that as many as one-fifth of all genes in our blood cells undergo seasonal changes.[1] The studies found that, in Europe and Oceania/Australia, places of middle latitude, the blood contains a denser blend of immune responders during winter. In summer, meanwhile, the blood increases in fat-burning, body-building, and water-retaining hormones. Further research needs to be done on populations living close to the equator and high latitudes, as they have very different seasons.

Much research also highlights that our molecular clock, our biological circadian rhythm (sleep-wake cycle), is impacted by environmental dysregulation. This occurs in heavily industrialised countries with long hours spent indoors, excessive artificial light, jet lag, night shift workers, and mothers with children who don't sleep. Disruption to our circadian rhythm prevents effective healing through DNA repair. It also disrupts the balance of important neurotransmitters, such as serotonin and melatonin, which are important for mood and body cycle regulation. The disruption of our circadian rhythm is detrimental to our health, resulting in increased rates of cancer, heart disease, and avoidable accidents.

It is better for our biological circadian and seasonal rhythms to be in sync with the natural light-dark cycles of our twenty-four-hour day. So, we need to get enough sleep when it is dark, get outside in natural light during the day, and pay attention to our surrounding environment. I encourage you to take time outside and observe nature. Do this for both for the nature recharge benefit and to synchronise with, rather than work against, your local seasons. The more we recognise and align with our local seasons and cycles the more balanced, healthy, grounded, and equanimous we feel.

I have partnered the five element seasons from TCM with the Eastern Kulin nation's seasonal calendar (see table 3.2).[2] The Kulin nation is an alliance of five Indigenous Australian nations in south central Victoria, Australia. I currently reside in Melbourne/Naarm and this lies on the land, seas, and waterways of the traditional custodians of the Boon Wurrung people of the Kulin nation. Their seasonal calendar is based on changes in the types of animals hunted, in the flowers and plants harvested, and in the stars and weather.

If you reside in a place of middle latitude and even some areas of low latitude, you can partner the five element seasons with your own local indigenous calendar. This can help guide you further with attuning to your surrounds and choosing self-care practices, as discussed further in this book.

Table 2.2. TCM's Five Element Seasons and the Eastern Kulin Nation's Seasonal Calendar

Australian Months	Five Element Seasonal Calendar	Eastern Kulin Nation Seasonal Calendar
January	Summer • *Fire* element is more vulnerable, attend to the Heart and Small Intestine • Hot weather • Growth • Red • Yang energy	Biderap (Dry) Season • Hot, dry weather • High temperatures and low rainfall • Bowat (Tussock) grass is long and dry • The Southern Cross is high in the south at sunrise • Female common brown butterflies are flying
February	Late Summer (last two weeks of February and first two weeks of March) • *Earth* element is more vulnerable, attend to Spleen and Stomach • Transformation • Yellow/Gold • Point of transition from yang to yin energy	Biderap
March	Autumn • *Metal* element is more vulnerable, attend to the Lung and Large Intestine • Harvest • White • Yin energy	Iuk (Eel) Season • Hot winds cease and temperatures cool • Iuk (eels) are fat and ready to harvest • Binap (Manna Gum) is flowering • Days and nights are equal length
April	Autumn	Waring (Wombat) Season • Cool, rainy days follow misty mornings • Highest rainfall and lowest temperatures • Waring (wombats) emerge to graze and bask in the sunshine • Days are short, and nights are long
May	Autumn	Waring
June	Winter • *Water* element is more vulnerable, attend to the Kidney and Urinary Bladder • Store • Black / Dark Blue • Yin energy	Waring
July	Winter	Waring
August	Winter (Early Spring) • Both *Water* and *Wood* elements are vulnerable, attend to the Kidney, Urinary Bladder, Liver, and Gall Bladder	Guling (Orchid) Season • The cold weather is coming to an end • Guling (orchids) and Muyan (Silver Wattles) are flowering
September	Spring • *Wood* element is more vulnerable, attend to the Liver and Gall Bladder • Birth, blossoms • Green • Yang energy	Poorneet (Tadpole) Season • Temperatures are rising, but the rain continues • Pied currawongs call loudly and often • Days and nights are equal length • Gurrborra (koalas) start mating, the males below at night • Tubers are ready for eating
October	Spring	Poorneet
November	Spring	Buath Gurru Grass (Kangaroo Grass) Flowering Season • The weather is warm • It is often raining • Buliyong (bats) are catching insects in flight
December	Summer • *Fire* element is more vulnerable, attend to the Heart and Small Intestine • Hot weather • Growth • Red • Yang energy	Gunyang (Kangaroo-Apple) Season • Changeable, warm, thundery weather • Dhuling (goannas) and buliyong (bats) are active • Bundjil (wedge-tailed eagles) are breeding • Days are long, and nights are short

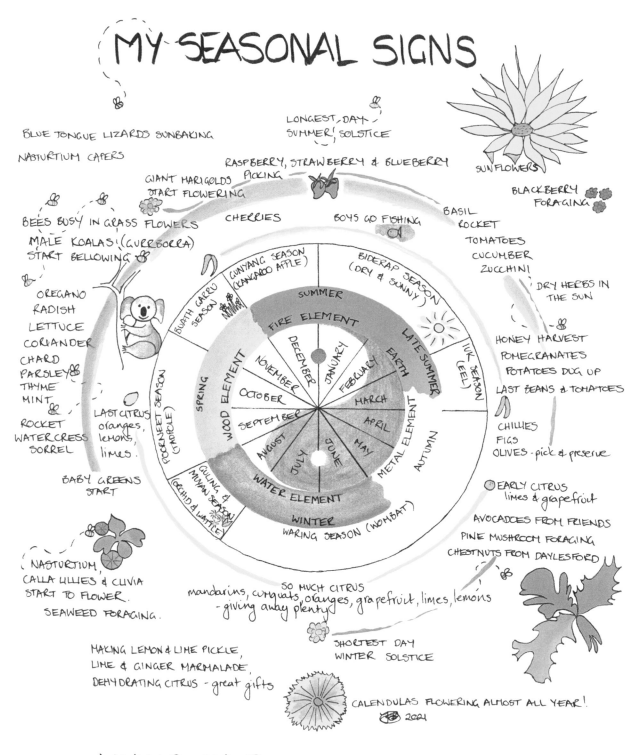

MY SEASONAL SIGNS

LIVING ON BOON WURRUNG COUNTRY
OF THE KULIN NATION

Reconnect with Nature

Do you make the time to notice your surrounding natural environment regularly? Do you have a park or body of water nearby? Or perhaps you have the blessing of a backyard or garden surrounding your home? Can you consciously dedicate five minutes a day to really become *aware* of your surrounding natural environment? When we spend time in nature, we become happier and healthier.

If you have the physical ability to move outside, then do. Go for a walk, shuffle, run, scoot, skip, skate, dance, or ride outside each day. Can you do this without headphones in your ears? Can you listen, look, smell, and even touch your surrounding natural environment? Immerse yourself. Open your senses to your natural surroundings and notice what season you are currently in. Reconnect to nature.

Five-Minute Nature Reconnect Practice

In this practice, I invite you to take a small moment of time to notice your surrounding natural environment—to really notice it, even if you live in a city.

To prepare for this practice, I invite you to go outside. Perhaps you can move out onto a balcony or a veranda, or even better, a backyard or nearby park or body of water. If you can't go outside, open a window and sit in front of it (or you can even do this short practice in the car with the window wound down).

Ring.

So, let's get our mindful bodies on. Bring yourself into the present moment by deliberately adopting an open and upright posture if you're sitting or standing. Or, if you're lying on your back, lie balanced and symmetrical with an open posture.

I invite you to take a deep belly breath (if you can), and gently lengthen your exhalation, to help calm your body and mind. (Inhale … exhale.)

I invite you now to close your eyes and take another deep breath. What can you smell? Notice any scents or aromas nearby? Notice with a gentle curiosity. What can you smell outside?

I invite you now to bring your attention to sounds. What can you hear outside? Perhaps you can hear the sound of birds, insects, people, traffic, wind in the trees, rain. Just listen with a gentle curiosity. Allow the sounds to help call you into the present moment.

I invite you now to bring your attention to touch. What temperature can you feel caressing your face? Or perhaps there is another area of your skin that is in direct contact with the outside. Is there a warm breeze? A cold biting wind? Is it still? Is it hot or cold? What temperature is it outside and how does it feel against your skin?

I invite you now to open your eyes and notice what you can see outside? Are there plants and trees nearby? What colour and shape are they? Are there flowers? Are there leaves? Can you see any animals, insects, or people? What is the quality of light like? Are there clouds in the sky? What colours can you see? Just look with a gentle curiosity. Cultivate a sense of wonder.

What season is it where you are?

As we come towards the end of this practice, I invite you to send some gratitude out to our precious planet and take a moment to realise and acknowledge the life-supporting connection we have. Take a conscious breath in and allow your heart to fill with gratitude. As you breathe out, send gratitude out to our precious planet. Give Mother Earth some deeply felt thanks.

Breath in… and out.

Ring.

I invite you to start to gently reactivate and re-energise your body with a deeper breath or two, perhaps a wriggle of the fingers and toes, or you might like a little stretch.

When you're ready, you can go on your way.

Thank you.

Nature Recharge

Nature recharge is the nickname I use for the positive mental, physical, and spiritual benefits accrued from time spent in nature. The natural world is such a powerful stress reliever and mood booster. There are so many lessons to be learnt by quietly observing and truly submerging yourself in nature. Have you experienced the power and magic of a nature recharge?

Australian indigenous people have appreciated the value of connecting to Country for millennia. They acknowledge the reciprocal relationship we have with Country. Country has cared for and healed First Nations people physically, spiritually, socially, emotionally, and culturally for thousands of years. In return, indigenous Australians listen deeply and respect and care for Country.

I often share this inspiring poem when discussing the magic of a nature recharge whilst teaching. It is written by Wendell Berry, a current, talented American poet, farmer, and environmentalist:

> *"The Peace of Wild Things"*
> *When despair for the world grows in me*
> *and I wake in the night with the least sound*
> *in fear of what my life and my children's lives may be,*
> *I go and lie down where the wood drake*
> *rests in his beauty on the water, and the great heron feeds.*
> *I come into the peace of wild things*
> *who do not tax their lives with forethought*
> *of grief. I come into the presence of still water.*
> *And I feel above me the day-blind stars*
> *waiting with their light. For a time*
> *I rest in the grace of the world, and am free.*[3]

Note: I encourage you to listen to Wendell reciting this poem; a recording can be found at https://onbeing.org/poetry/the-peace-of-wild-things/.

Nature Recharge Guidance

1. Find an area of nature and wild things. This may involve a body of water, a forest, an expanse of wide-open space, or mountains.

2. When you arrive, please take a deep breath and set your intention for practice. Acknowledge Country, the land, or the body of water you are submerged in:

   > "I vow now to cultivate mindful attention towards this precious place, this place of nature and wild things.★ I will use my senses to tune in and reconnect. I will explore slowly with respect, grace, and a gentle curiosity. I will allow any feelings to arise, paying particular attention to calm, wonder, and awe."

3. Begin to move slowly and silently. Notice your surroundings. Listen. Smell. Feel. See. Breathe. Make friends with the natural world. Cultivate awareness.

4. If you start to feel distracted by a stream of thought, or if you feel rushed, just gently slow down or stop. Feel your feet on the ground (or in the water). What can you hear? What can you see? What can you smell? What can you touch? How do you feel?

5. Find a comfortable place to be still. Rest here for a while (fifteen to twenty minutes).

6. As you come towards the end of your nature recharge, I invite you to take a moment to send some gratitude out to our precious planet. Realise and acknowledge the life-supporting connection we have. Take a conscious breath in and allow your heart to fill with gratitude. As you breathe out, send gratitude to our precious planet. Give Country / Mother Nature some deeply felt thanks.

★If you know the ancient or indigenous name for this area or place, please insert it here. If you know of the ancient custodians of the land, seas, and waterways on which you recharge, please also pay your respects to them.

If we all start to reconnect to our natural environment and its wild things, then we can heal both ourselves and our precious planet. Here I share an inspiring excerpt from the book *Braiding Sweetgrass* by Robin Wall Kimmerer.[4] She writes with such beauty and wisdom. I found her whole book to read like one long gentle and wise poem: "For all of us, becoming indigenous to a place means living as if your children's future mattered, to take care of the land as if our lives, both material and spiritual, depended on it."

This is something we can all work towards, becoming indigenous to the place on which we reside.

Chapter 3
Helpful Stress and Unhelpful Stress

Stress and Our Nervous System

Stress is defined as an organism's total response (physical, chemical, and emotional) to change and/or pressure. We can have healthy stress and unhealthy stress.

When does stress become harmful and unhealthy? When discussing the positive and negative effects of stress, we need to understand our nervous system. Here is a brief introduction.

Our nervous system is made up of our brain, spinal cord, and nerves. It controls and coordinates most of our body through electrical and chemical means. It reacts to changes (stressors) both inside and outside of the body.

Within the brain, we have our limbic system. This system is involved in our behavioural and emotional responses. There is a small almond-shaped part of our limbic system called the amygdala. Our amygdala switches into action when it thinks we are in danger or under threat. Unfortunately, the amygdala is unable to tell the difference between a real threat (for example, an oncoming car) and a perceived threat (for example, watching an action-packed movie or the news). Whatever the cause, once something has been interpreted as a threat, our hypothalamic-pituitary-adrenal (HPA) axis is triggered.

Our HPA axis releases stress hormones into the bloodstream and activates our sympathetic nervous system (SNS). When the SNS is activated, our thinking becomes fear based and/or goal oriented, and our bodies power up with strength, speed, and focus. More blood is directed to our limbs and hindbrain. This is called the "fight-flight" response, also known as the "stress response." It primes our body, ready to fight or flee, freeze, please, or faint. It allows us to protect ourselves from threatening situations or manage challenging situations.

Our autonomic nervous system (ANS) acts largely unconsciously (automatically). It is composed of our SNS and parasympathetic nervous system (PNS). It regulates our heart rate, digestion, respiratory rate, pupillary response, urination, and sexual arousal.

Our PNS is composed mainly of the cranial nerves, including the vagus nerve and sacral spinal nerves. Its main function is to activate the "rest-digest" response, also known as the "relaxation response." It causes more blood to flow to our digestive system and our organs. It helps our body rest and return to homeostasis following a fight-flight response. It triggers our body into "rest, digest, heal and grow mode."

PERIPHERAL AUTONOMIC NERVOUS SYSTEM

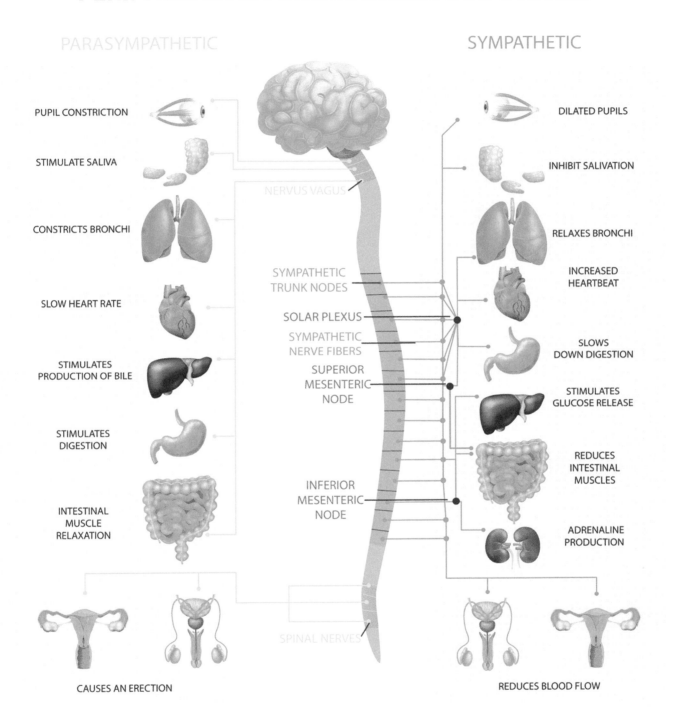

PARASYMPATHETIC

SYMPATHETIC

PUPIL CONSTRICTION

STIMULATE SALIVA

NERVUS VAGUS

CONSTRICTS BRONCHI

SLOW HEART RATE

STIMULATES
PRODUCTION OF BILE

STIMULATES
DIGESTION

INTESTINAL
MUSCLE
RELAXATION

SYMPATHETIC
TRUNK NODES

SOLAR PLEXUS

SYMPATHETIC
NERVE FIBERS

SUPERIOR
MESENTERIC
NODE

INFERIOR
MESENTERIC
NODE

SPINAL NERVES

DILATED PUPILS

INHIBIT SALIVATION

RELAXES BRONCHI

INCREASED
HEARTBEAT

SLOWS
DOWN DIGESTION

STIMULATES
GLUCOSE RELEASE

REDUCES
INTESTINAL
MUSCLES

ADRENALINE
PRODUCTION

CAUSES AN ERECTION

REDUCES BLOOD FLOW

MAINTAINS HOMEOSTASIS

MOBILIZES RESERVES
UNDER STRESS

Table 3.1. Active Parasympathetic Nervous System versus Active Sympathetic Nervous System

	Active Parasympathetic Nervous System	Active Sympathetic Nervous System
Physical Response	• Decreased muscle tension • Increased serotonin & melatonin • Reduced heart rate & blood pressure • Increased diaphragmatic breathing • Improved digestion & nutrient absorption • Balanced immune function • Increased tissue & cell repair • Reduced pain • Increased alkalinity & oxygenation • Sensitisation • Sensuality	• Hyperactive amygdala (threat detector) • Increased muscle tension • Increased cortisol & noradrenalin • Increased heart rate & blood pressure • Increased shallow, costal breathing • Decreased digestive enzymes, food absorption & waste elimination • Immune system deregulation • Decreased cell & tissue repair; decreased healing • Increased acidity & toxicity • Increased sense of pain but general desensitisation • Increased free radicals & inflammation • Increased cholesterol & fats in bloodstream • Increased shortening of telomeres & genetic instability • Increased tumour angiogenesis
Mental Response	• Rest • Fun & enthusiasm • Increased attention & memory • Nurturing & healing • Open awareness & presence • Increased growth & interaction • Greater sense of empathy & connection • Increased vitality • Intuition • Patient	• Hyperarousal, hypervigilance • Excess busyness, constant doing • Excess thinking that can't be switched off • Narrow focus of attention • Excess control • Excess goal orientation • The "more syndrome" (always needing more) • Excess judgement • Emotional reactivity • Defensive • Impatient
Mode	Rest, digest, heal and grow	Fight, flight, freeze and please
	Flow	*Contraction*

Short-Term versus Long-Term Stress

Our modern way of living, fast paced and overstimulated, often results in chronic stress. This is long-term, low-grade, ongoing stress. There are constant demands and pressures. We are often go, go, going or do, do, doing. We are programmed to always achieve and/or constantly please. There is little time for, or approval of, rest and relaxation. This results in long-term activation of the HPA axis, leading to deregulation and pathology. This is unhelpful stress.

We also have our own individual variances of the fight-flight response to consider. This is influenced by early life events, current lifestyle, genetics, age, and gender. Research (and hundreds of years of experience!) show that our female hormones make us even more vulnerable to stress. Women are at twice the risk of developing stress-related diseases such as depression; anxiety; fibromyalgia; IBS; and autoimmune diseases like Hashimoto's disease, diabetes, and multiple sclerosis. So, as women, we have even more reason to pour into our cup and activate our PNS.

Table 3.2. Short–Term and Long–Term Stress

Short-Term Stress / Acute Stress:	Long-Term / Chronic Stress
• Protects us from threatening situations, such as dealing with an oncoming car accident, a fight, and so on • Helps us deal with challenging situations, such as meeting a deadline, competing in sports events, taking a test, delivering a presentation • Turbo charges us, resulting in our being productive, focused, attentive, and motivated	• Involves chronic over-activation of the SNS without sufficient rest or relaxation • Can be caused by ongoing pressures and demands such as always being on the go, always planning, always achieving, continuous problem solving, and constantly pleasing or rescuing others • Gradually results in physiological wear and tear on our body, commonly seen in chronic depression and anxiety, which occurs more commonly in females • Can become a habitual way of being, we can become addicted to the adrenaline rush, and it becomes the "normal" way of life • Can be influenced by external circumstances, social conditioning, family patterns, insecurities, and past trauma
Short term stress is healthy, normal, natural and necessary	*Long term stress is a health risk*

Chapter 4
Self-Care

You can't pour from an empty cup. Take care of yourself first.

—Author unknown

Self-care as a woman—what does this look like for you?

Let's first start with defining what self-care is in this book, as there can be a blurry line between self-care and indulgence. Self-care is our individual cultivation of kindness and methods of care towards ourselves. The purpose of self-care is to maintain our health and well-being. It includes positive lifestyle choices and taking responsibility for ourselves.

Do you treat yourself with kindness? Can you offer yourself comfort and empathy when times are tough? Do you have boundaries in place? Can you treat yourself as you would a small innocent child or a good friend, with unconditional love, particularly when times are tough?

Remember we all have both good and bad days. We can all experience harsh and judgmental thoughts inside our head. These can be exacerbated by childhood conditioning, photo-shopped social media and marketing campaigns, hormones, and our gut health. Recognising and acknowledging that thoughts are just thoughts, not truth, can help lead us to the road of kindness and true self-care.

I will be sharing practices and methods of self-care for women in this book. We will discuss mindful movement and exercise, mindful eating, and mindful meditation in detail. The importance of sleep, true rest, keeping hydrated, and knowing your menstrual cycle are also discussed. Please remember we are all individuals, so our self-care practices will be too.

Self-care is so important, yet it can be difficult to prioritise in a modern world that values constant hard work and productivity. Please remember self-care is *not* selfish. How can your body operate well without giving it the time, space, and appropriate support to rest and heal? How can you be there for others and love others fully if you can't be there for yourself or fully love yourself? How can you truly help others if you can't accept or ask for help for yourself?

As a health practitioner, a teacher, a patient and a friend, I have seen many women with only a few drops left in their cup. Add the magic of motherhood into the equation, and self-care can get really tricky. Ultimately, we are all responsible for our own health and well-being; we know our body better than anyone else if we take the time to listen and learn from it when we are of sound mind. It is important to recruit help when we need it, but please remember that, generally, it is best if we are the CEO of our own health and self-care.

By tuning in to the cycles of nature and through certain self-care practices, we can begin to hear the voice of our own inner feminine nature. This is our intuition. When we combine our intuition with science and reason, we can gain a broader perspective and often make better decisions. For true self-care, we need to reconnect to our intuition.

In the words of Lao Tzu, "The power of intuitive understanding will protect you from harm until the end of your days."[1]

When we make the opportunity to pause, tune in, make our heart sing, and harmonise with our environment, we are filling our cup. When we pour into our cup and take care of ourselves, we can then be the mother, grandmother, friend, partner, sister and young girl we truly are, within our heart.

Mindfulness

When first introducing the definition of mindfulness whilst teaching adults and children, I ask them to pay attention to this cup.

This cup was introduced to me by my friend and teacher Janet Etty-Leal. She was at the forefront of teaching mindfulness to children in Melbourne over twenty years ago.

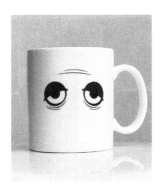

I ask students "How do you think this cup is feeling right now?"

Their replies are usually, "tired, sad, sleepy, down, empty."

I then pour hot water into the cup and ask them to watch carefully. The cup changes. "Now how do you think this cup is feeling?"

Their replies are usually, "happier, full, *awake*." Awake is the key word that I am looking for.

Mindfulness is waking up to the present moment, to what you are experiencing right now, both within and around you. Importantly, it is doing so with an attitude of kindness, with an open heart, and with a gentle curiosity. When we wake up and pay attention, the world fills us with wonder.

There has been a surge in research over the last decade into mindfulness and its positive impact on our physical and mental well-being. It has been shown to improve brain function in areas related to executive functioning, attention control, self-regulation, sensory processing, memory, and regulation of the fight-flight response.

Mindfulness is simple but not easy. It is a skill, like many, that develops with practice.

There are both formal and informal forms of mindfulness. An example of an informal mindful moment is when you are completely absorbed in the beauty of an ocean sunset. You can smell the tang of the ocean and the seaweed. You can hear the sound of the waves and the birds calling. You can feel a warm breeze caressing your skin and the soft sand between your toes. You can see the golden glow of colour permeating the sky. All your senses are immersed in this present moment. Your heart feels expansive and full.

We all experience moments of mindfulness, but they are often fleeting. The busier we become the less often informal mindful moments occur. The frenetic pace of our modern lifestyle often leaves us incapable of appreciating the subtle, gentle, and wondrous things in life. Throughout *Wonder Full Women*, I have included boxes with suggested formal mindful meditation practices. We have already explored a formal "Five-Minute Nature Reconnect Practice." We will also explore mindful movement and mindful eating in detail in the next few chapters. The gift of wonder depends on mindfulness, humility, and gratitude. We will work on cultivating all three of these during the seasonal practices shared in this book.

As G. K. Chesterton wrote in *Tremendous Trifles*, "The world will never starve for want of wonders; but only for want of wonder."[2]

Compassion and Loving-Kindness

Compassion is being aware of pain and suffering, coupled with the wish and effort to alleviate it. Compassion connects feelings of empathy to acts of kindness and generosity.

"Compassion is the wish for another being to be free from suffering; love is wanting them to have happiness." This was shared by His Holiness the Fourteenth Dalai Lama (HHDL), the spiritual leader of the Tibetan people and of Tibetan Buddhism. He has been promoting the message of kindness and compassion for decades and was awarded a Nobel Peace Prize for doing so in 1989.

True compassion is unconditional—it is kindness and support offered without anything expected in return. True compassionate action feels wholehearted, spontaneous, and natural. It warms our heart. There is no underlying resentment or expectation.

Women, in general, are conditioned and expected to be "nice" and offer constant kindness and support to others. It can be this conditioning that leads to burnout and poor health, particularly if our own needs are unmet, unseen, or unheard. When women (and men) go out of their way for others but have no kindness towards themselves and have little or no self-compassion, this results in a lack of healthy boundaries, and their cups are easily emptied.

As defined by Kristen Neff, a leader in teaching self-compassion in the United States of America, self-compassion involves self-kindness, a sense of common humanity and mindfulness.[3]

Self-kindness involves treating ourselves with care and understanding, rather than harsh and critical judgement. When we practise kindness towards ourselves, genuine kindness towards others grows. As our own well-being

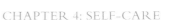

increases, we are then able and likely to be more patient, supportive, forgiving, and loving. To take care of others, we have to take care of ourselves; otherwise, we start running on empty. Just like the safety demonstration at the start of an air flight tells us, we have to attend to our own oxygen mask first before we can safely help others. As our happiness and other inner strengths grow, we then have more to genuinely offer others.

Gaining a sense of common humanity involves seeing our position with a wider perspective and becoming aware of being part of a larger human experience. Life can be hard. When we resist life's hardship, it intensifies our suffering. We then have two causes of suffering. We suffer not only because it is painful in the moment, but also because we are resisting and banging our head against the wall of reality. We get frustrated because things are not how we would like them to be. What we resist persists.

Mindfulness, as we discussed above, involves "being" with the present moment, including the painful feelings. Our brains are wired to feel the emotions of others through our mirror neurons. This means that, when we are in the presence of people in pain or suffering, we also feel that pain or suffering in our own brains. So, it is absolutely crucial to learn how to validate and give compassion to ourselves, particularly for those of us who are caregivers.

There is a yin and yang aspect of self-compassion. The yin involves being there for ourselves. It involves comforting, soothing, and validating ourselves. This includes speaking to ourselves with kind words and thoughts, not as harsh critics. It includes giving ourselves a hug when needed or the gift of time to take a long, warm, soothing bath full of Epsom salts.

The yang of self-compassion involves positive action, such as protecting, providing, and motivating ourselves. It includes knowing our limitations and putting boundaries in place. It includes knowing when and how to say no. It also involves actively doing things to look after ourselves, such as eating well, drinking enough water, and getting enough sleep.

Here are some guided meditation practices to help build and strengthen compassion.

A Mindful Moment with Kind Thoughts for Kids (and Adults)

So, let's get our mindful bodies on. Sit open and upright, still and strong like a mountain. Or perhaps you are lying on your back, balanced and symmetrical.

Palms are open and resting on your lap or resting over your belly or resting by your side.

Please close or lower your eyes.

Ring.

Start with three delicious, deep belly breaths to help calm your body and mind and activate your parasympathetic nervous system.

Breathing in … breathing out … breathing in … breathing out … breathing in … breathing out. Just let your breath settle now; let your breath breathe you.

Shift your focus now to the sound of the bowl. *Ring.* Listen until you can no longer hear it ring. (Pause.)

Let's finish our mindful moment with some kind thoughts. So, as you breathe in, say silently in your mind, *May I be well and happy.* And as you breathe out, *May others be well and happy.*

You might like to picture in your mind your friends or family, a group, or an individual on your out breath and picture yourself on your in breath.

Breathing in, *May I be well and happy.*

Breathing out, *May others be well and happy.*

Breathing in, *May I be well and happy.*

Breathing out, *May others be well and happy.*

When you're ready, you can open your eyes.

Thank *you.*

Loving-Kindness Practice for All

So, let's get our mindful bodies on.

Take a moment to adjust your posture.

If you're sitting, sit open and upright like a mountain. Or if you're lying down, lie balanced and symmetrical with legs out long. Or you may like to bend and support your knees to take pressure off your lower back.

Palms are open and resting by your side, on your lap, or over your belly.

If you haven't already done so, please close your eyes.

I invite you to take a wide face-stretching yawn, with an audible release on your exhalation. Allow all the muscles of the face to soften.

Draw your shoulders blades in and down your spine. Open your heart space.

Just settle into your body. Perhaps taking three slow, deep belly breaths helps.

Allow your body to relax and release on your exhalation. Relax and let go that little bit more with each exhalation. (Pause.)

Ring … relaxing, awake, and alert.

Remember, there is nothing you need to be doing right now. There is nothing you need to experience or achieve during this meditation practice. This is your time.

Allow your breath to find its own depth and rhythm now; just let your breath breathe you.

I invite you now to bring your attention to the **s***pace in front of your eyes*. It's like a field of darkness. Perhaps there are some muted shapes or colours there, but we're not looking for anything; we're simply resting our attention here, in this space, with relaxed eyes and a soft gaze. (Pause.)

I invite you now to bring your attention to any *sounds* coming from outside the room. Just listen with a gentle curiosity.

Allow the sounds to come and go without resistance.

Now bring your attention to sounds inside the room. Just listening without judgement. Perhaps you can notice the sound of your own breath, your digestion, even your heartbeat.

Allow the sounds to call you into the present moment, just listening. (Pause.)

I invite you to draw your attention further to your *breath*. Begin to notice any sensations associated with your breath as you breathe in and as you breathe out.

Can you feel the slight movement of your chest and your belly?

Can you feel the air flowing past your nostrils?

Just follow each breath. Let your breath breathe you.

Allow your breath to help anchor you into the present moment. (Pause.)

I'm going to share some phrases, and I invite you to gather your attention behind each phrase, one at a time. You don't have to try to fabricate or manufacture any special feeling. But, rather, shepherd your attention back to the following phrases. Be as completely present behind each phrase as you can be. If you ever find your attention has wandered, don't judge yourself; just gently and kindly bring your attention back to each phrase and your breath.

I invite you now to bring to mind yourself.

Breathe in. Consciously direct the breath to your heart, wish yourself well, and say silently in your mind:

May I be filled with loving-kindness.

May I treat myself with kindness in good times and in hard times.

May I be peaceful and at ease.

May I be well. May I be happy.

Breathe in and allow your heart to fill with loving-kindness. Breathe out and send loving-kindness out to every part of your being. (Pause.)

I invite you now to bring to mind someone you love. Visualise a child, a pet, a good friend, or your partner this time—just one person. You are going to wish them well.

Breathe in, consciously direct the breath to your heart, and say silently in your mind:

May you be filled with loving-kindness.

May you treat yourself with kindness in good times and in hard times.

May you be peaceful and at ease.

May you be well. May you be happy.

Breathe in and allow your heart to fill with loving-kindness. Breathe out and send loving-kindness to this loved one. (Pause.)

I invite you now to take this beautiful feeling you have for the people you love and spread it across to somebody you don't know so well. Picture in your mind a neutral person. You might choose a neighbour, your postman, or a shopkeeper. Visualise this person.

Again, direct the breath to your heart and say silently in your mind:

May you be filled with loving-kindness.

May you treat yourself with kindness in good times and in hard times.

May you be peaceful and at ease.

May you be well. May you be happy.

Breathe in and allow your heart to fill with loving-kindness. Breathe out and send loving-kindness to this person. (Pause.)

I invite you now to picture in your mind someone you find difficult to love—perhaps someone who has hurt or disappointed you. If you are just beginning with this practice, please start with someone who has hurt you just a little, not too much. We are going to try and remember that they too want to be happy, just like us. Visualise this person.

Breathe in, consciously direct the breath to your heart, and try to wish this person well by saying silently in your mind:

May you be filled with loving-kindness.

May you treat yourself with kindness in good times and in hard times.

May you be peaceful and at ease.

May you be well. May you be happy.

Breathe in and allow your heart to fill with loving-kindness. Breathe out and send loving-kindness to this person. (Pause.)

Now I invite you to join me in wishing all beings loving-kindness; you might like to rest your open palms over your heart.

Again, starting with ourselves, visualise yourself and say silently to yourself, *May I be well and happy.*

Visualise your family. *May my family be well and happy.*

Now visualise your friends. *May my friends be well and happy.*

May everyone in our local community be well and happy.

May everyone in this country be well and happy.

May all beings, all over the world, be well and happy. May all beings enjoy true peace. May we all be filled with loving-kindness and appreciate this one wild and precious life. May we be filled with grace and gratitude.

Just rest for a few moments in the feeling of loving-kindness as it spreads. Allow that warm, fuzzy feeling to fill your heart and flow out to every cell of your body. Allow it to flow out to all beings. (Long pause.)

Ring.

I invite you now to slowly start to reactivate and re-energise your body. Perhaps take a deeper breath or two. Wriggle your fingers and toes. You might like to have a little stretch. Give yourself a hug.

Thank you.

In my summary of compassion, I offer you another two quotes to consider—one from my son, shared when he was aged four, and one from the spiritual director and co-founder of FPMT (the Foundation for the Preservation of the Mahayana Buddhist Tradition):

> *"Mum, love is the best, love is good … 'cause if we didn't have love imagine what would happen if a little baby came out of its mummy's tummy and there was no love?!…The baby would just be lost." —Zachary*

> *"Compassion is the most important practice in life." —Lama Zopa Rinpoche*

Befriend Your Body

Just like when I spend time in nature, when I spend quality time with my body, I am left with feelings of wonder and awe. Our bodies are complex and magical. They are able to heal. In the first twenty-four months of our lives, we experience incredible growth and development of our bodies. And the fact that most women can create and birth another human is extraordinary.

It can be hard befriending our body in the modern world. Constant marketing campaigns and the media often leave us feeling ugly, flawed, weak, fat, not enough, and on and on. Throughout this book, we will share practices to cultivate kindness, respect, and wonder for our female bodies, particularly during the mindful movement practices. These latter practices provide us with a way to reconnect and listen to our bodies.

We want to work *with* our bodies, not against them. What we resist persists. Rather than pushing, ignoring, or changing our bodies in forceful ways, we want to work respectfully with our bodies, including our heart and mind. We want to respect and nurture ourselves in tune with our surrounding environment and its seasonal and cyclical changes.

Despite the many years of scientific research into the intricacies of how our bodies work, there is still much that is unknown. There are similarities yet differences between individuals. Let us combine science, along with our own self-awareness and intuition. This way, we can find the most individual and beneficial self-care practices for ourselves.

In the words of Jo Phee, "We cannot heal what we cannot feel."[4]

Female Cycles and Seasons

Women experience menstrual cycles and body seasons. By body seasons, I am referring to our different life stages—birth, childhood, puberty, adult, perimenopause, menopause, death.

For those of you with a menstrual cycle, do you know the patterns of your cycle? Keeping a record can help, either via a paper diary, or there are some great apps out now. You can track your period's start and end date, along with signs and symptoms (such as breast tenderness, mood, energy levels, and digestion). Our hormones impact our internal world and how we live in the external world. So, by becoming friends with your cycle, you can begin to harmonise with your body, rather than working against or ignoring it. Keeping a record of your cycle can also offer you a helpful account of what is happening with your health in general.

Remember that stress can impact our menstrual cycle. It can inhibit our reproductive system and stop ovulation and menstruation (secondary amenorrhea). I have personally experienced this, most noticeably when I moved countries. And I have also seen and helped many women with secondary amenorrhea whilst working as a health practitioner.

Your cycle length is the amount of time / number of days from the start of one period to your next period. Day one of your cycle is the first day of your period when you experience significant blood loss. As women, our cycle lengths vary. The female cycle can vary from twenty-four to up to thirty-six days, and that's OK.

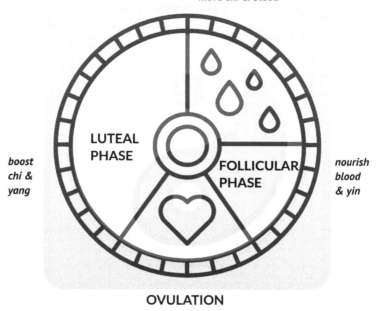

MENSTRUATION
move chi & blood

LUTEAL
PHASE

boost chi & yang

FOLLICULAR
PHASE

nourish blood & yin

OVULATION
move chi & blood, strengthen yang

Yin and Yang of the Menstrual Cycle

Phase 1: Menstruation

During the first few days of your bleed, your hormones are low, and so is your energy. This is a time to rest and spend time alone or with the people you love. Gentle exercise only. Don't take on anything extra and, if possible, clear your diary.

Phase 2: Follicular Phase / Pre-Ovulation

Your oestrogen starts to increase, and so does your energy. Maisie Hill, author of *Period Power*, fabulously describes oestrogen as your Beyonce hormone—outgoing, sassy, energetic, and flirty. Oestrogen wants you to get out in the world (and find someone to reproduce with). This is the time of your cycle when you feel like Wonder Woman. It is a good time to get creative, start new projects, exercise vigorously, and have sex. Your yin (feminine) energy is building.

Phase 3: Ovulation/Transition

Luteinising hormone surges and triggers the release of an egg. In TCM, your yin energy peaks with ovulation. This is a time to verbalise your thoughts and feelings and engage in creativity.

Phase 4: Luteal Phase / Post-Ovulation

Once you ovulate, your oestrogen decreases, and you can find yourself lacking in motivation and starting to feel depleted. Self-doubt can creep in, so this is not a time to make big decisions. Where on earth did Wonder Woman go?! For some women, this feels like a sudden change; for others, it can be more gradual. As your progesterone increases, you often feel like slowing down. Your metabolism increases (so you feel hungrier), and it's a time to prioritise sleep. In TCM, yang energy increases, particularly if the egg is fertilised and you become pregnant. There is a lot of energy required for the rapid cell division involved in growing a baby. The few days before your period is due is a time to hibernate and increase self-compassion and self-care; this applies if you are pregnant or not.

MENSTRUAL CYCLE

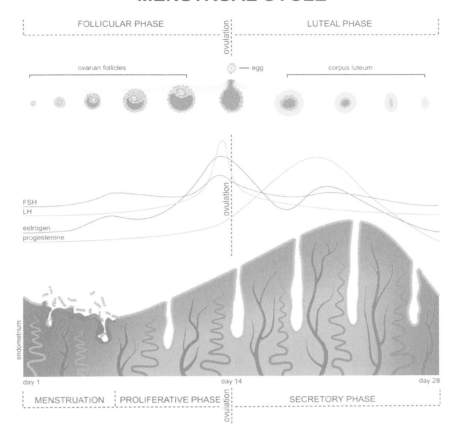

Being aware of these natural shifts in hormones, energy, and metabolism can help us to work *with* each menstrual cycle, rather than against it. If you know your oestrogen is increasing (during the proliferative phase of follicular phase), then this is a time when you will enjoy socialising and "getting shit done." On the other hand, during the week or so before your period is due (luteal phase), your energy will start to wane. This is a time to slow down, clear your calendar of meetings, and minimise socialising. It's time to increase gentle self-care practices instead.

Perimenopause refers to the life season or phase that occurs anywhere from two to twelve years before menopause. Your actual cycle may still be regular. Yet hormonal changes may result in symptoms such as hot flushes, changes to menstrual flow, feelings of rage, fatigue, brain fog, poor memory, and insomnia. It is a season in your life when it really helps to be prepared and informed.

The average age for the onset of menopause is anywhere from forty-five to fifty-five years old. Menopause is the cessation of menstruation. It is the life season or phase that begins one year after your last period.

So, where you are in your life seasons will affect you physically, chemically (hormonally), and emotionally. Tuning in to your body and befriending it can help all these changes flow more smoothly (pun intended).

If you would like further information on navigating your hormones and attuning to your life seasons and cycles, I highly recommend Maisie Hill's two books *Period Power* and *Perimenopause Power*, along with her podcast (further details can be found in the resource section of this book).

What Makes Your Heart Sing?

What makes your heart sing? What makes you feel alive and fills your cup? What nourishes your soul?

I invite you to take some time to sit down for ten to fifteen minutes and really have a think about what personally nourishes your soul and makes your heart sing. Write out twenty or more big and/or small things that you know nourish your soul and make your heart sing. You can then go back and look at this list or add to it, whenever you need inspiration.

I've shared my list below, in the hope it may help give you some inspiration.

Freya's Heart Sing List (in no particular order)

- Daily meditation (this is non-negotiable for me)
- Ethically sourced cacao, a natural heart opener
- A heartfelt hug
- Mindful movement—dance, yoga, chi gong, playing with inversions on the FeetUp Trainer
- A meal made with love and seasonal foods; relaxed dining plus stimulating conversation
- Sharing grateful things each day with my boys
- Being kind to myself, noticing when I am not (noticing negative self-talk and gently and/or humourously redirecting it)
- A nourishing conversation with a friend
- Walking and noticing my surrounding environment
- Singing along loudly to a favourite song
- Giving myself time to be creative—pottery, writing, cooking, doodling, painting, drumming (I find creativity helps quieten my over-analytical and judgmental thinking mind.)
- Gardening, picking home-grown goodies, and eating them
- Swapping home-grown goodies with friends and neighbours
- Spending time in Somers (a small coastal town in Victoria) (Do you have a "happy and healing" place?)
- Piecing together a puzzle
- Allowing myself time to read nourishing and enriching words
- Both practising and teaching mindfulness, meditation, and yoga
- Home-made "life-changing sourdough crumpets" (recipe found in *Grown & Gathered*, details in bibliography) with my chocolate hazelnut spread (detailed in "A Little Extra" chapter)
- Watching the sunrise or sunset
- Cuddles with Louis (our cat)
- Connecting and spending quality time with my husband, our boys, and/or good friends
- An art gallery visit
- Time in nature
- Laughing
- Genuinely helping others

Can you incorporate at least three things that make your heart sing into each day?

Gratitude

Scientists have discovered that our brains have a "negativity basis." This means our brains tend to ruminate and dwell on the "bad things." So bad news sticks to us like Velcro, and good news slides right off us like a Teflon non-stick pan. Thankfully, scientists have also discovered that our brains are neuroplastic. This means they can change. Just like our muscles, the more we use our brain in a certain way (the more we fire neurons in a certain way) the stronger those neuronal pathways build. We can think of it like a dirt road transforming into a freeway due to regular use. Have you heard the saying "neurons that fire together wire together"? If we use our brains often in positive ways and take the time to relish the good, then our brains will rewire towards feeling happier and calmer.

Examples of positive ways to use our brain are practising gratitude daily, pausing to relish positive moments, calming ourselves with belly breathing, daily meditation, being kind to ourselves and others, doing things that make our heart sing, and laughing lots.

Gratitude humbles the thinking mind and activates positive neuroplasticity. It can be a healing force. Research has found that gratitude is associated with greater spiritual well-being. It expands and nourishes our heart. I have personally found a regular gratitude practice to be healing for myself and my family.

Cultivating gratitude into each day can be simple.

Ways to Cultivate Gratitude

- Share three grateful things around the dinner table each night.
- Keep a gratitude jar. Each day during the week, family members or close friends can write down their grateful things on a piece of paper and add it to the jar. At the end of the week, everyone can read and share the grateful things together.
- Acknowledge three grateful things just before bed or first thing in the morning; either share them with another person or write them down in a diary.
- The What's Good App is another way to record your three grateful things daily. Each day, the app provides a new inspiring quote, a beautiful photo of nature, and the opportunity for you to write down your three grateful things. The app records and stores your grateful things, and you can return and reflect on them at any time.

"Impermanence, the Dalai Lama reminds us, is the nature of life. All things are slipping away, and there is a real danger of wasting our precious human life. Gratitude helps us catalogue, celebrate, and rejoice in each day and each moment before they slip through the vanishing hourglass of experience."[5]

A Mindful Moment with Gratitude for Kids (and Adults)

Ring.

So, let's get our mindful bodies on, sitting open and upright like a mountain or lying down on your back, balanced and symmetrical, still and quiet, palms open and resting in your lap or over your belly or by your side. Please close or lower your eyes.

Take three delicious, deep belly breaths to help relax and calm your body. Breathing in … breathing out … breathing in … breathing out … breathing in … breathing out. Just let your breath settle. Just let your breath breathe you.

Listen to the sound of the bowl until you can no longer hear it ring. *Ring.* (Pause.)

Now picture in your mind three big things you are grateful for—perhaps it is your home, your family, a pet, a teacher. Whilst picturing these three big things in your mind, place a hand over your heart and say silently to yourself, *Thank you, thank you very much.* Breathe in and let your heart fill with gratitude. Breathe out and let that warm, fuzzy feeling flow through your whole body now.

Now picture in your mind three small things that you are grateful for, things that you often forget about or take for granted—it might be the warm sun on your face, a hug from a friend, a smile, your clothes, your hands, your breakfast. Whilst picturing these three small things in your mind, keep your hand over your heart and say silently to yourself, *Thank you, thank you very much.* Breathe in and let your heart fill with gratitude. Breathe out and let that warm, fuzzy feeling flow through your whole body.

Just take a moment now to notice how you feel after relishing and thanking these things you are grateful for. Do you feel happier?

Remembering to feel grateful about the big and the little things in your life can be really helpful.

Next time you're feeling sad, angry, lonely, or afraid, see if you can think of three things you feel grateful for and then notice how you feel.

Ring.

As we come towards the end of this mindful moment with gratitude, you might like to wriggle your fingers and toes, have a little stretch, and then open your eyes when you're ready.

Thank you.

There are some longer, more detailed recordings of my guided gratitude practices on Insight Timer—"The Gratitude Practice" and "Gratitude Practice during Covid-19."

Chapter 5
Move with the Seasons

"Wild Geese"

You do not have to be good.
You do not have to walk on your knees
for a hundred miles through the desert, repenting.
You only have to let the soft animal of your body
love what it loves.
Tell me about despair, yours, and I will tell you mine.
Meanwhile the world goes on. (emphasis mine)

—Mary Oliver

Note: I encourage you to view the full poem and listen to Mary reciting this poem; a recording can be found on the Best Poems Encyclopedia website at https://www.best-poems.net/mary_oliver/wild_geese.html.

Mindful Movement

Our body loves our attention. It wants to communicate and work with us. We are often so caught up in our "head," in our busy yang world, that we end up disconnected from our bodies—that is, unless our body starts to communicate loudly, perhaps even scream at us with a health crisis.

Mindful movement is when you engage with your body whilst it moves. Attention is consciously directed towards the sensations associated with the movement of your body and its breath. It involves tuning into your sense organs—external (exteroception) and internal (interoception). External senses are based on our eyes, ears, skin, and nose—what we can see, hear, feel/touch, and smell. Our internal senses include our vestibular system (our sense of balance), spatial orientation, proprioception (sense of body position), and nociception (sense of pain).

Learning to slow down, focus, and practise forms of mindful movement can help us to reconnect to our body and our intuition. There is wisdom in our body that we can benefit from. Well-known forms of mindful movement, many of which have been practised for centuries, are yoga, tai chi, martial arts, qi gong, and dance. I am grateful to have experience with most of these forms of mindful movement. Practising mindful movement is a way to incorporate more yin into our busy yang lives. For the last five years, I have found yin yoga and inversions particularly helpful and healing. We will explore these two in further detail.

Many people find it hard and uncomfortable to drop into a meditation practice, with their minds too busy with thoughts. Traditionally yoga asana was used to help prepare for meditation. Mindful movement performed prior to meditation can help calm and settle your mind. Do you have any favourite forms of mindful movement that help you to reconnect to your body and its breath?

Please note that most movement can be mindful, providing you focus your attention on the body with its sensations, along with your surroundings in the present moment. Running, walking, and even playing a musical instrument can all be a form of mindful movement. Finding balance with our choice of movement and exercise, both yin and yang, is important for our health.

When we first bring attention to our body sensations, they can be quite dull. We may not be able to feel or notice much. With time and practice, we begin to feel more subtle and strong sensations. When we direct our attention towards our sensory perception of our body and its breath, our thinking mind goes offline. We can let go of the unconscious stream of thought with its endless to-do lists and drop into the present moment. Our mind calms down. Our PNS is activated so our rest, digest, heal, and grow mode is online. As a result, the health of both our body and our mind improves.

Contemplative practices, such as mindful movement and meditation, restore a person's sense of presence and agency in the world.[1] By regularly practising and cultivating awareness of our body sensations, our heart, and our mind, we develop our presence and a wider perspective. This allows us to find purpose. It allows us to adapt and navigate the roller coaster of life with greater ease.

Fascia

Let us explore fascia, in the context of the human body, to help us appreciate mindful movement further.

As described by the Fascia Research Congress, fascia is a sheath, or sheet of connective tissue that forms to attach, enclose, and separate muscles and other internal organs.[2] Our fascial system is a collagenous connective tissue network that runs throughout the whole body and holds all our cells together. It weaves our muscles and bones together. It holds our organs in place.

We have differing areas of fascial density throughout the body. Our cartilage, ligaments, and tendons are thick, dense areas of fascia. Our muscles are sheathed and infused with a cotton candy like net of fascia.

Fascia is not inert. It has the ability to move, stretch, and recoil. It is elastic, which means it has the ability to resist a distorting influence (a stretch, squash, or squeeze) and then return to its original size and shape. If we avoid stretching and stressing any of our tissues, including our fascia, we invite atrophy (a slow steady decay of the tissues abilities). If we do not stress our fascia, our joints tighten up, and we lose range of motion. But overstretching is also a concern. So, what is a healthy amount of stress/stretch? We will discuss this further in the yin yoga section.

There is more and more research and development occurring in the field of fascia. Some scientists are now describing fascia as a delivery system, like the nervous system and circulatory system. It is rich in nerve endings important for proprioception and interoception (the sense of our internal body state).

The Fascia Research Congress defines the fascial system as a "three-dimensional continuum of soft, collagen containing, loose and dense fibrous connective tissues that permeate the body … The fascial system surrounds, interweaves between, and interpenetrates all organs, muscles, bones and nerve fibres, endowing the body with a functional structure, and providing an environment that enables all body systems to operate in an integrated manner."[3]

The healthy movement of our fascia is impacted by:
• Scar tissue
• Surgery
• Age
• Inflammation
• Fluid metabolism
• Habitual posture

Yin Yoga

Yin yoga is a slow, nourishing, and healing form of yoga. It incorporates principles of TCM with hatha yoga poses/asanas. The asanas are held for longer periods of time than in other yoga styles, anywhere from two to ten minutes. Most asanas are held on the floor, and props can be used for extra support if required. Yin yoga primarily impacts our fascia, rather than our muscles. Our muscles are activated in more yang/active yoga styles. Yin yoga impacts the deep fascial network of our joints, ligaments, tendons and even our bones.

Specific sequences of yin asanas can be created with the intention of impacting certain TCM meridians. We will explore this further in the individual asana descriptions and individual season chapters.

Some studies suggest that these long held, less intense asanas can squash or squeeze water, metabolic waste, and inflammatory waste products out of the area(s) targeted. The moderate stress to the fascia also stimulates strengthening of the joints and helps to remove blockages/adhesions. Flexibility and circulation to the joints is improved.

The mental component of learning to hold each asana for a longer period of time is a practice in patience. We also learn to breathe and relax into a little discomfort. Over time, the practice of relaxing into discomfort can result in less reactivity in everyday life.

The "rebound" is the period of rest, in a comfortable position, following the yin asana. The rebound allows chi/prana/energy to flow through the body more freely following the long-held asana.

During each long-held asana and rebound, we tune into the sensations of our body and our breath. This sharpens our sense of interoception. We also cultivate a gentle curiosity towards any feelings and thoughts as they arise. This all helps to calm the mind and cultivate an ideal attitude for a longer mindful meditation practice.

"Although the challenge of being still seems to stem from physical discomfort, for most people, it is predominantly a mental issue. Learning to open to difficulty without resistance is the domain of mindfulness training and is a highly practical and liberating tool for life. The Yin poses (more so than the Yang) can be a viable way to begin a meditation practice, helping us slowly become more comfortable in our bodies and minds." This is an excerpt from *Insight Yoga* by Sarah Powers, another of my esteemed teachers.[4]

Four Principles to Guide Us in Our Yin Practice

1. Come into the pose

Come into the selected asana and find your appropriate edge. This can also be called your "sweet spot" or "Goldilocks position." This is where you feel the body being stretched, squashed, or squeezed not too little, not too much, but just right.

We find our appropriate edge by slowly coming to a point of resistance and then pausing. Tune in to your body and notice how it feels. Can you feel a significant stretch, squash, or squeeze? There will be some discomfort. Feel into and direct attention towards the target area(s) described. We need to listen and learn to tell the difference between risky pain and discomfort. If you begin to feel overwhelmed or alarmed; your breath becomes restricted or fast; you sense sharp, shooting, stabbing pain or strong burning, electrical tingling sensations, these are all signs of risky pain. You need to consciously come out of the asana immediately and modify. Please make sure you are physically safe in each asana.

Don't concern yourself with how you *look* in the pose; it is how you *feel* in the pose that's important. I find remembering and sharing the following anonymous quote found in Bernie Clark's book *The Complete Guide to Yin Yoga* very helpful: "We don't use the body to get into the pose, we use the pose to get into the body."[5]

How you feel in the asana is much more important than how you look. Due to normal individual anatomical variation, we can all look quite different in a pose, despite targeting the same area(s). I offer a few physical variations of each asana to accommodate anatomical variation in chapter 7 of this book.

Bernie Clark offers a wonderful website resource, found at www.yinyoga.com. It lists all the yin yoga asanas and their variations. He has also written *Your Body, Your Yoga*, which explains, in great detail, all the ways in which normal anatomical variation influences our ability to move and perform certain asanas.

2. Surrender

Once you have found your Goldilocks position, become still and mentally willing to surrender to the experience. Stillness of the body leads to a quieting of the breath and, in turn, the mind. Turn "yinside," as phrased by my teacher Jo Phee.[6]

3. Marinate

Allow your body the time to ferment and marinate in each asana. Choose to stay in the asana for a while (anywhere from two to five minutes is common). Decide on the length of time you plan to hold each asana at the beginning of your practice. The only reason to modify your pose is to either shift a little deeper into it or come out of it. Reasons to come out of the asana are pain you deem risky or a sense of overwhelm.

When moving out of the asana use breath awareness and move *slowly*. Please be aware that immediately following a long-held yin asana, our joints can feel quite fragile and vulnerable; this feeling is normal and should pass after a minute or two whilst you rebound.

4. Rebound

The rebound is where the magic happens. Choose a position of comfort for your rebound (options are shown in chapter 7 of this book). Whilst in this position of comfort, notice the echo of the previous asana. Can you feel a warmth, tingling, vibration, or an increased flow of blood and/or energy spreading out from the targeted area(s)? One of my dear clients describes the rebound feeling like a gentle internal shower—like a gentle warm fluid feeling flowing and washing through the inside of her body.

The rebound can be experienced in three ways—physically, emotionally, and mentally. Physically, you may experience a warmth, vibration, tingling, and/or physical sense of ease. Emotionally, you may experience a release, perhaps with tears of grief or feelings of anger arising. Mentally, you may experience memories arising, thoughts of gratitude, insights into the future, creative flow and/or a "light bulb moment." (Our creativity flows when our PNS is stimulated.)

Val's Story

Val first started coming to my adult meditation classes in 2017 and has been practising with me since then. I have Val to thank for encouraging me to start teaching adult classes (to not only teach at schools), and she has been a strong advocate for my classes, workshops, and retreats since. When I started incorporating mindful movement into my adult classes in 2018, Val shared that she finds the mindful movement an important key to help her access her meditation practice.

I have such a busy mind that it is too big a leap to drop straight into a seated meditation for me. I find the mindful movement, along with your verbal prompts of directing our attention towards our body sensations and breath, helps me transition to a slower pace of mind. The mindful movement is an essential intermediary phase for me. It prepares me for our meditation practice ... I also find the power of group practice takes you to a different level, a higher level, versus a solo practice.

—Val

Inversions

In relation to mindful movement, an inversion is defined as any pose or movement that aligns our heart above our head. Inversions have been practised for thousands of years.

There are yang versions and yin versions of inversions. Some yang inversion examples are handstand (*Adho Mukha Vrksana*), forearm stand (*Pincha Mayurasana*), and supported headstand (*Urdhva Dhanurasana*). Some yin inversion examples are Wall Caterpillar (*Viparita Karani*) and Happy Baby (*Ananda Balasana*), which can be found in detail in Chapter 6.

It is important to remember that inversions aren't appropriate for everyone. There are contraindications and cautions, particularly for the more yang inversions.

Contraindications to yang inversions:
- Glaucoma
- Retinal detachment
- Eye issues/infection
- Recent stroke, brain injury, or concussion

Cautions for yang inversions:
- Unmedicated high blood pressure
- Low blood pressure (Make sure you come out of any inversion very slowly.)
- Shoulder issues (Monitor the comfort of your shoulders.)
- Current headache (The increase in blood flow to the head can increase headache intensity.)
- Current head infection (sinusitis, ear infection, and so on) (The increased blood flow to the head can be very uncomfortable.)
- Perimenopause/menopause (It can trigger a hot flush.)
- Heavy period
- Heart conditions
- Pregnancy
- Recent Botox injections
- Recent surgery

If you're unsure about inverting, please discuss it with your health practitioner. Do a little research for yourself, both academic as well as experiential. Remember, if at any stage you feel uncomfortable in any pose or something doesn't feel right, please carefully come out of the pose. You know your body better than anyone else. Listen to your body.

The Wonderful Benefits of Inversions

1. Improved blood flow to head and brain, which helps with concentration and memory
2. Improved lymph flow, which can help increase immunity
3. Help with digestion and detoxification
4. Relief of excess fluid build-up in the legs
5. Help building core and upper body strength
6. Increased energy
7. Help in building confidence (the more yang versions)
8. Ability to have a new perspective on life
9. Awakening of the playfulness and fun of our inner child
10. Longevity.

One of my esteemed teachers, Dustin Brown, introduced me to the FeetUp Trainer in early 2019. It has allowed me to slowly increase my core and arm strength and to be able to incorporate more yang style inversions back into my daily practice. I really appreciate how these yang inversions provide me with a shift in perspective, allowing my heart to align above my head, both physically and mentally. The increased blood flow to my brain helps to heal my nervous system. I find it great for my overall health, energy, and mental clarity. I always feel a lightness in my heart, a bounce in my step, and a playful attitude following the use of my FeetUp Trainer.[7]

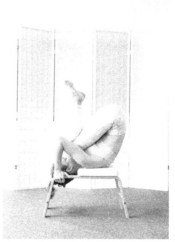

Rock and Roll

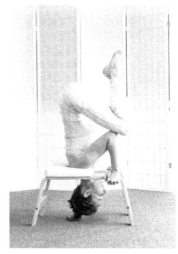

The Gift

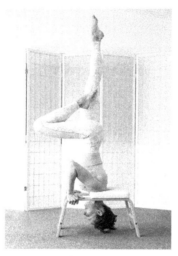

One Leg

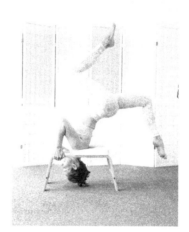

Dropping Back

Meridian Tapping

When we tap along external meridians (we can't tap along the internal branches, as they run inside the body), we can impact chi flow. Tapping the body along the natural direction of chi flow, along each meridian, is toning and stimulating.

For more delicate areas, such as the face, use the tips of your fingers to tap. You can use cupped hands along arms, torso, and legs. There are contraindications to meridian tapping. Avoid the initial meridian tapping step in each seasonal practice (found in Part II of this book) if any of these contraindications or cautions apply to you. Please check with your trusted health practitioner to clarify your individual situation.

Contraindications for meridian tapping:
- First three months of pregnancy
- Low back and sacral area tapping during entire pregnancy
- When you have a fever
- If you have any infectious skin disease or illness

Cautions for meridian tapping:
- Osteoporosis, tap gently
- When you are feeling extremely anxious or nervous, it may be too stimulating
- Heart conditions
- Any conditions where you have an increased tendency to bleed, tap gently

Chapter 6
Asana and Pranayama

Pranayama

Prana is a Sanskrit word that translates as "life force." *Ayama* translates as "to expand" (different to *yama*, which translates as "to restrain or control"). *Pranayama* is the practice of focusing on and altering our breath, in such a way that the prana is freed, expands. or extends. It helps to calm and steady our mind, so it is a helpful prelude to meditation.

There are many types of pranayama. The following three styles are the ones I share regularly in my classes. There are many more advanced breath practices, which require more in-depth in-person teaching.

Belly Breath

Otherwise known as diaphragmatic breath, belly breathing involves taking slow, smooth breaths. Newborn babies breathe this way.

Belly breathing steps:

1. Take a slow breath in through the nose, directing the breath down into your belly.
2. Allow your belly to gently expand like a balloon, slowly counting to four. (This is not always easy if you are new to belly breathing. With practice, it will get easier.)
3. Pause.
4. Exhale slowly and allow your belly to deflate like a balloon, slowly deflating to the count of four.
5. Pause. Then begin again.

When I teach this type of breathing to primary school kids, we first make an origami boat. We also discuss chest breathing, where the breath is high up in our chest and belly breathing, where the breath is low in our belly:

Chest Breath = Stressed Breath (easy to remember because it rhymes), our sympathetic nervous system is active.

Belly Breath = Calming Breath, our parasympathetic nervous system is active.

Once the excitement of boat building has settled, we all lie down on our backs and place our boat over our belly button. It is helpful to prop our heads up with a pillow or place our arms under our head, and then we are able to watch the boat with a relaxed neck. We practise rocking our boat with our belly breaths.

The more we formally practise belly breathing, the easier it is to use at other times of the day when we want to calm down. I also direct belly breathing throughout my mindful movement and meditation classes.

I've used mindful belly breaths in a fight where I breathed and said I'm sorry.

—E, year 3

You help me go to sleep better and I can get less angry because I take three deep belly breaths.

—G, year 3

Thank you for teaching me to be more calm and take deep belly breaths like when my sister fights me I don't fight back. I be calm and feel like she never did it.

—Lulu, year 3

Long Exhale Breath

Long exhale breath builds on slow belly breathing.

Long exhale breath steps:

1. Once you feel comfortable with your belly breathing, begin to consciously lengthen your exhalation.
2. As you come towards the end of your exhalation, activate your lower abdominal muscles and pelvic floor, activate your *mula bandha* (root lock), to help expel the last amount of air.
3. Start by lengthening your exhalation by a count of two; inhale for six and exhale for eight. Work towards inhaling for a count of six and exhaling for a count of twelve. Some people like to breathe in and out through the nose, some like to inhale through the nose and exhale through the mouth; either option is fine.

When I teach this breath practice to kids, we breathe out long through the mouth, and it is called "Blowing Out the Birthday Candles Breath."

There has been recent research into the breathing techniques used in contemplative practice (for example meditation, yoga, tai chi). In 2018, Roderick Gerritsen and Guido Band of Leiden University in the Netherlands published a detailed theoretical review that presented a wide range of studies.[1] These studies all illustrate how slower respiration rates and longer exhalations stimulate the vagus nerve. This means they activate our PNS into rest, digest, heal, and grow mode.

As Gerritsen and Band put it, "Frequently adopting these respiration patterns (slowed and with longer exhalations) can explain a significant part of the efficacy found within contemplative activity practice. Though contemplative activities are diverse, they have shown a similar pattern of beneficial effects on health, mental health, and cognition: mostly in stress-related conditions and performance. This pattern can be explained by these controlled breathing exercises."[2]

Ujjayi Breath

The *ujjayi* breath is also known as the victorious breath or oceanic breath. It is said to sound like waves rolling up against the shore. It strengthens our respiratory system, lungs, and diaphragm. It also helps to relieve constipation. It is particularly helpful during autumn but can be used at any time of the year.

It involves the long, slow breaths that activate our parasympathetic nervous system. Thus, our relaxation response is activated. The mind begins to calm down, which helps quieten any unconscious striving and/or aggressive feelings. This in turn can help to prevent injuries during asana practice.

You can use ujjayi breath throughout your asana practice, or you may like to use a few ujjayi breaths in preparation for your meditation practice.

Learning How to Ujjayi Breathe:

1. When first learning how to ujjayi breathe, start in a seated position with your spine long and your hands resting over your lower belly.
2. Inhale through your nose, mouth closed. As you exhale, consciously draw your belly back towards your spine, activate your mula bandha by lifting through your pelvic floor and contracting your lower abdominal muscles.
3. Inhale with your mouth closed. Exhale with your mouth open, whilst continuing to activate your mula bandha; whisper the word "whisper", extending the "r" sound as you do so. Can you notice the slight constriction at the back of the throat? This helps to slow and lengthen your breath.

---

4. Inhale with your mouth closed. Start exhaling with an open mouth whilst making an "r" sound and halfway through, close your mouth whilst continuing the "r" sound.

5. Now, with your mouth closed and the back of your throat slightly constricted, take an equal length inhalation and exhalation, slowly breathe in and out for four to six seconds each.

Note: It is easier for most beginners to constrict the back of the throat on exhalation. Keep practising and, before you know it, you will be making sounds like waves rolling up against the shore.

Yin Asanas

Ankle Stretch

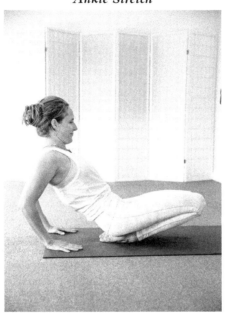

Target area:
- ▷ Stretches along the front of the ankles
- ▷ Stimulates meridians in the feet; Stomach, Spleen, Urinary Bladder, Kidney, Gall Bladder and Liver

Practising the pose:
- ▷ Begin by sitting on your heels with hands resting on your knees. Sit upright. This may be enough of a stretch for you.
- ▷ To increase sensation, lean back with hands still on knees or with palms placed behind you.

Hold time:
- ▷ Thirty seconds to one minute (depending on tolerance)

Caution:
- ▷ Knee issues, ankle issues
- ▷ Avoid or attempt very carefully if you have past ankle and/or toe fractures

Props:
- ▷ You may like to place a pillow or folded blanket under your feet for extra cushioning if your ankles are sensitive.

Bananasana

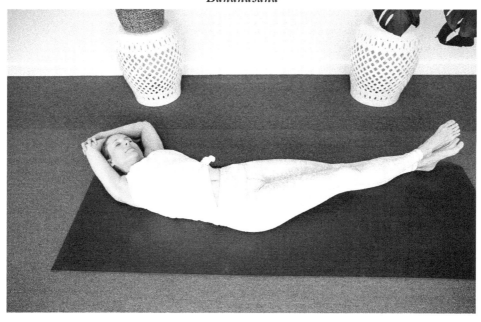

Target area:
- ▷ Stretches along one side of the body and into the shoulder, whilst squashing/compressing the opposite side.
- ▷ Stretches along the Gall Bladder meridian.
- ▷ With arms up overhead, it also stretches along the Heart, Small Intestine, Pericardium, and Triple Warmer meridians.

Practising the pose:
- ▷ Start lying on your back with your legs mat-width apart. Take a breath in and lift your right leg up and take it over towards the left. You may like to rest the right ankle on top of or underneath the left ankle.
- ▷ Keep your pelvis in the centre of the mat and start to shift your shoulders and upper torso over towards the left side of the mat, so you are making a banana shape.
- ▷ Lastly, bring your arms up overhead. Be particularly careful or avoid this step if you have any current or past shoulder injury. Hold onto your right elbow, right forearm, or right wrist to help increase the stretch along the right side of your body.
- ▷ Feel into the stretch along the right side of the body. You are creating more space for the right lung lobes and other organs lying along the right side of the torso.
- ▷ Allow the right side of your ribcage to gently expand on your inhalation, allow fresh oxygen to enter down into the right lower lung lobes.
- ▷ To come out of the pose, first release the arms on an exhalation and return them to your side. Next, gently shift your torso and shoulders back to lie in the middle of the mat. Lastly, release your legs so they are resting evenly on the mat.
- ▷ Rebound for thirty to sixty seconds in Constructive Rest Pose (CRP) or Savasana before swapping sides.

Hold time:
- ▷ Three to five minutes

Caution:
- ▷ Past or current shoulder injury

Prop options:
- ▷ You might like to place a small pillow or blanket under the head and/or shoulder.

Butterfly

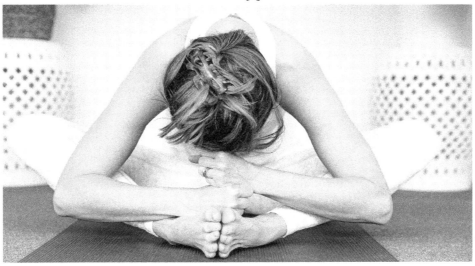

Target area:
- ▷ Stretches the lower back, hips, and groin
- ▷ If your head is rolled forward, it also stretches along the spine
- ▷ Stretches along the Gall Bladder, Urinary Bladder, Kidney, and Liver meridians

Practising the pose:
- ▷ From a seated position, bend your knees and bring the soles of your feet together.
- ▷ Round your spine and fold forward (see variations if your neck or low back are felling vulnerable).
- ▷ Allow gravity to pull the knees downwards and open the hips. Relax and let go a little more with each exhalation.
- ▷ To come out of the pose slowly roll your spine back upright and gently straighten your legs. Take a full inhalation and exhalation to do this.

Hold time:
- ▷ Three to five minutes

Caution:
- ▷ Can aggravate sciatica.
- ▷ Do not draw the soles of your feet too close to your groin in a yin seated Butterfly. Keep legs loose.
- ▷ Keep an upright seated position or choose Wall Butterfly or Reclining Butterfly if your neck or low back are feeling vulnerable.

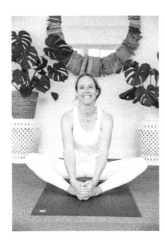 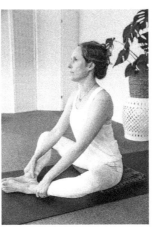

Prop options:
- ▷ You may like to sit on top of a small pillow or folded blanket to help elevate and tilt the pelvis forward.
- ▷ You may like to rest your head on a block or two or rest your chin on your hands with your elbows resting on your legs or the floor.
- ▷ You may like to place support, like a block or bolster, under the bent knees.
- ▷ You may like to wrap a blanket around your ankles for cushioning if they feel tender resting on the floor.
- ▷ You may like to place a block between your feet.

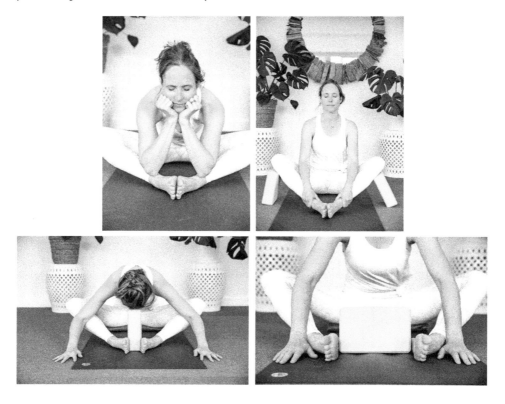

Variations:

Half Butterfly
- ▷ One leg is bent; the other leg is out long.
- ▷ You will be stretching along the hamstring of the straight leg.
- ▷ Individual hip anatomy impacts this pose. You may prefer to cross your bent leg over the top of your straight leg (this is called half shoelace) or if you naturally have more internally rotated hips, you may prefer to bend your leg in a Half Frog position (see Frog).

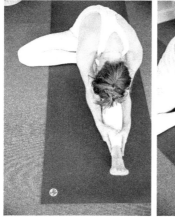
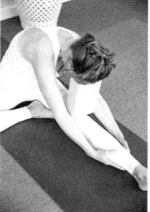
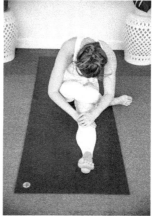

Reclining Butterfly
▷ Rather than rounding your spine and folding forward, recline backwards and rest your torso on the mat or a bolster.

Wall Butterfly
▷ Place your mat perpendicular to a wall. Start with your torso lying on the mat and rest your legs up the wall (see Wall Caterpillar). Bend your knees and bring the soles of your feet together.
▷ Your feet will align closer to the groin in Wall Butterfly.

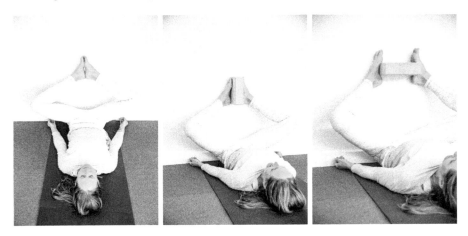

Cat Pulling Its Tail

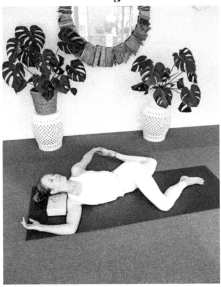

Target area:
▷ Stretches along the front of the lower hip, the lower hip flexor muscles, and quadriceps
▷ Stretches and opens the upper shoulder and arm
▷ Twists through the spine and gently compresses the lower back
▷ Stimulates the Stomach, Spleen, Liver, and Kidney meridians with the twist through the torso
▷ Lung, Large Intestine, Heart, Small Intestine, Pericardium, and Triple Warmer meridians are stretched along the top arm

Practising the pose:
▷ Start from lying on your right side with your knees and elbows bent 90 degrees and stacked in front of you.
▷ Slide your bottom leg (right) behind you. Bring your right heel towards your buttocks.

▷ Lift your top arm (left) and place your left hand to rest on your left hip with your elbow dropped back. *Or* you may be able to reach back and hold onto your tail (your right foot).

▷ You can increase the stretch by looking behind you, towards your tail (your rear foot).

▷ Feel into the twist through the spine and lower abdominal organs. Feel the stretch along the front of the right thigh and hip.

▷ To come out of the pose, gently release the hold on your tail, and bring your top arm forward to stack your elbows again. Slowly draw the bottom leg forward to stack your knees together again.

▷ Rebound side-lying and then swap sides.

Hold time:

▷ Three to five minutes

Caution:

▷ If you have any low back and/or shoulder issues ease into the pose very gently, listen to your body, and modify or back out if needed.

Prop options:

▷ Block or pillow to support your head.

▷ If you can't hold onto your tail and you would like to increase your stretch, you may find using a strap helpful. Loop it around your shoulder and tail.

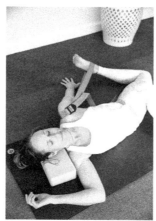 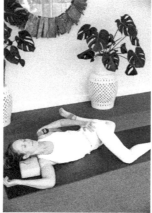

Caterpillar

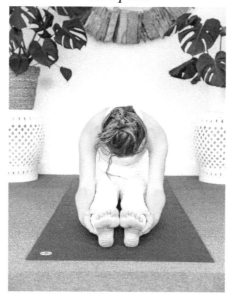

Target area:
   ▷ Stretches the hamstrings when the pelvis is tilted forwards
   ▷ Stretches along the back of the spine when the pelvis is tilted backwards
   ▷ Stretches along the Urinary Bladder meridian
   ▷ Gently squashes the lower torso organs

Practising the pose:
   ▷ Start seated with your legs out in front of you. Slowly roll your spine and fold forward.
   ▷ Feel the stretch along both hamstrings and along your spine.
   ▷ You can slightly vary the stretch by the tilt of your pelvis. The hamstring stretch is increased with your pelvis tilted forwards; the stretch along the back of your spine is increased when you tilt your pelvis backwards.
   ▷ Please bend your knees if your hamstrings are very tight. You may also need to widen the legs a little if you are experiencing any compression at the front of the hips.
   ▷ To come out of the pose, slowly roll back up to an upright position, stacking each vertebra as you go.
   ▷ Rebound seated.

Note: Paul Grilley says this is an excellent pose for balancing chi flow and preparing for meditation.

Hold time:
   ▷ Three to five minutes

Caution:
   ▷ Low back issues, sciatica.
   ▷ Widen legs if pregnant to allow space for the belly.

Prop options:
   ▷ Bend the knees and place a bolster under them for support (this will increase the stretch along the back of the spine).
   ▷ Place a bolster out long in between the legs with legs a little apart. This can help some people access folding forward.
   ▷ Support head with bolster or block.
   ▷ You might like to sit up on a cushion to elevate hips and pelvis, allowing them to tilt forward. This will increase the stretch through the hamstrings.
   ▷ If you experience hip compression, widen the legs a little or place a bolster or rolled blanket over the top of the thighs and lift your torso over the bolster/blanket before lowering your torso towards the legs. Or choose Dragonfly pose instead.

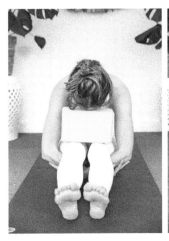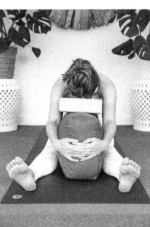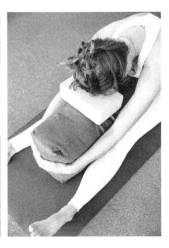

Variation:

Wall Caterpillar
 ▷ If your hamstrings are particularly tight, you might like to place a pillow under your pelvis; you can also move your pelvis away from the wall a little.
 ▷ Arms can rest by your side, over your belly, or over your head.

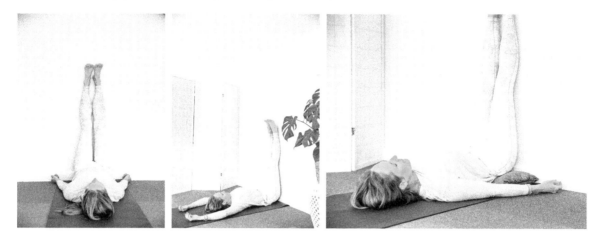

Child's Pose

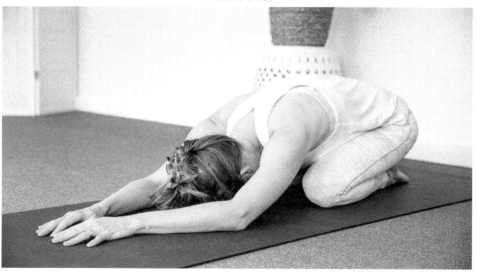

Target area:
 ▷ Stretches along the back of the spine
 ▷ Stretches the Urinary Bladder meridian
 ▷ Gently compresses the Stomach, Spleen, Kidney, and Liver meridians
 ▷ Side stretch version stretches the Gall Bladder, Heart, Small Intestine, Pericardium, and Triple Warmer meridians
 ▷ Wide knee version deeply stretches along the Liver and Kidney meridians running through the inner thighs
 ▷ Wide knee with twist version stretches and twists the Stomach, Spleen, Liver, Kidney, Large Intestine, and Small Intestine meridians.

Practising the pose:
 ▷ From all fours, gently push your hips back towards your heels and lower your head towards the floor.
 ▷ Your arms can rest long above your head, down by your side, or bent and stacked to offer a headrest.

- ▷ Widening the legs a little can help some people access folding forward more easily.
- ▷ This is a healing and soothing pose if you are feeling cold, anxious, exhausted, or vulnerable.
- ▷ To come out of the pose, slowly roll back upwards to an upright position, stacking each vertebra one at a time.

Hold time:
- ▷ Three to five minutes

Caution:
- ▷ Widen knees if pregnant to allow space for the belly.
- ▷ If you have just eaten, this pose may create uncomfortable pressure on your digestive system.

Prop options:
- ▷ You might like to support your head with a pillow or block or rest your head on your stacked forearms resting on the floor in front of you.
- ▷ If you have tight ankles and/or knees, you might like to place a pillow under the ankles and/or under or behind the knees.
- ▷ You might like to place a bolster under your chest.

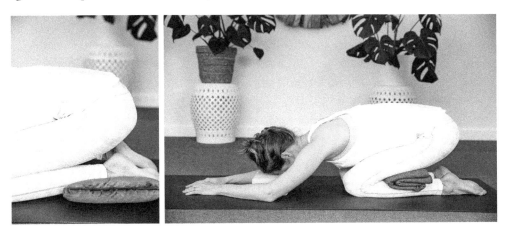

Variations:

Child's Pose with Side Stretch
- ▷ From Child's Pose with arms out long, slowly start to finger walk the hands towards the left side.
- ▷ Feel into the stretch along the right side of the torso, right shoulder, and along the right outer arm. Hold for one to two minutes.
- ▷ Swap sides by finger walking the hands to the right side.

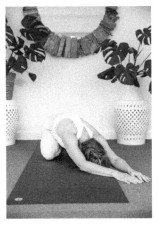

Wide Knee Child's Pose

  ▷ Widen your knee position in child's pose.
  ▷ Feel the stretch in the inner thighs and groin.

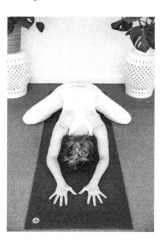

Wide Knee Child's Pose with Twist

  ▷ From Wide Knee Child's Pose, thread your right arm under your left.
  ▷ Place your right arm and shoulder onto the mat, making sure you have space between your right shoulder and upper neck/ear.
  ▷ You may like to use a block/pillow for head support and/or a blanket for knee cushioning.
  ▷ Rest your left hand on the floor, your left thigh, your sacrum, or all the way around to your right inner groin. Your hand position impacts the amount of twist through your spine and torso.
  ▷ Feel into the twist through the torso, the squeeze through the abdominal organs, the stretch along inner thighs, and the stretch along the back of the right arm.

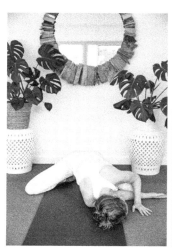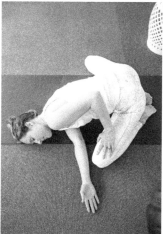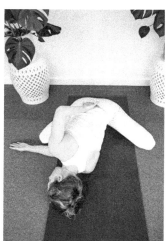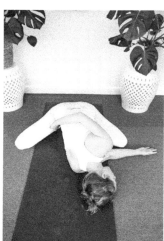

Deer Pose

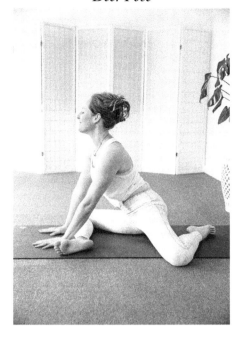

Target area:
  ▷ Stretches the thighs and hips
  ▷ A balance of hip rotation—forward leg has hip externally rotated; back leg has hip internally rotated
  ▷ Stretches along the Gall Bladder meridian
  ▷ With reclining twisted deer variation, it also stretches Liver, Kidney, Stomach. and Spleen meridians.
  ▷ With arm overhead, it also stretches along Heart and Small Intestine meridians.

Practising the pose:
  ▷ Start seated in Butterfly and then swing your left leg behind you.
  ▷ Try making a right angle with your front knee.
  ▷ Feel into your hips and thighs.
  ▷ Lean on to your hands to come out of the pose. You may like to gently windscreen wipe your knees before swapping sides.

Hold time:
  ▷ Three to five minutes each side.

Caution:
  ▷ Be careful if you have any knee issues. Try keeping the feet closer to the groin or opt for a different pose.

Prop options:
  ▷ If your knees are sensitive, try placing a blanket under them.

Variation:

Reclining Twisted Deer
  ▷ Snuggle a bolster up against your forward leg side of the pelvis. Breathe in, lift, and twist though your torso.
  ▷ Breathe out and drape your torso over the bolster.
  ▷ You can bring your arm above to increase stretch along the top of your torso, upper shoulder, and arm.

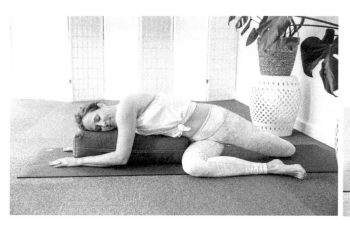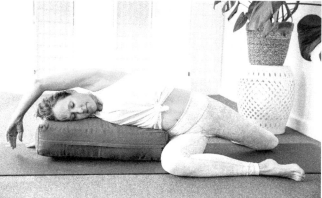

Dragonfly / Straddle

Target area:
- ▷ Stretches the inner groin, hamstrings, and hips
- ▷ Stretches along the Liver, Gall Bladder, Kidney, and Urinary Bladder meridians

Practising the pose:
- ▷ Start seated with your legs out long in front of you.
- ▷ Widen your legs and then slowly roll your spine to fold forward.
- ▷ Feel into the stretch along the inner legs.

Hold time:
- ▷ Two to five minutes

Caution:
- ▷ If you have any low back or neck issues, keep your spine straight. You may like to place your palms down on the floor behind your hips and press downwards to help increase sensation and stretch in the pose.
- ▷ If you have knee issues, do not widen the legs too far apart. You can also tighten your quadriceps, tighten the muscles around your knee joint.
- ▷ If your hamstrings and spine feel tight/stiff, you can bend your knees.

Prop options:
- ▷ Sitting on a small cushion will help tilt the pelvis forward. Be careful though; this can also increase knee hyperextension, in which case you can place a blanket or pillows underneath/behind the knees for support.
- ▷ You may like to place a bolster lengthwise between your legs and fold forward onto it for support.

Variation:

Wall Dragonfly
- ▷ From Wall Caterpillar slowly widen the legs.
- ▷ If sensation is too much, you can place your hands on the outer side of your thighs to help take some of your leg weight, or you can use a strap around your ankles.
- ▷ If you want to increase stretch and sensation, then you can place your hands on your inner thighs.

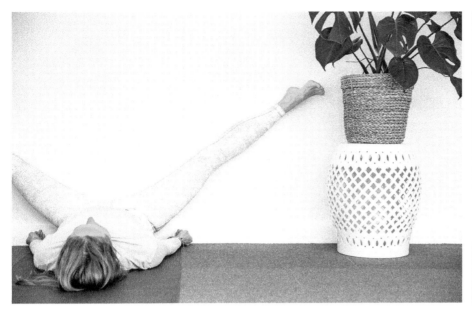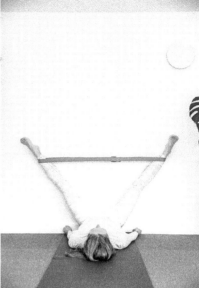

Dragons

Target area:
- ▷ Stretches along the front of the hips, thighs, and deeply into the groin
- ▷ Stretches along the front of the torso (particularly high dragon)
- ▷ Stretches along the Stomach, Spleen, Liver, Gall Bladder, and Kidney meridians

Practising the pose:
- ▷ From all fours, step your right leg forward. With your right knee bent place your right foot between your hands. Keep your hands on the floor.
- ▷ Gently slide and straighten your left leg out behind you.
- ▷ Hold. Feel into the stretch along the front of the left hip and thigh.
- ▷ Slowly release out of the pose by shifting your weight backwards and straightening out the right leg.
- ▷ Rebound with lengthening of the right leg, offering a gentle hamstring stretch.
- ▷ Swap sides.

Hold times:
- ▷ One to two minutes for each variation. Cycle through the chosen variations on each side before swapping to have the left leg forward.

Caution:
- ▷ If your body is feeling stiff, your back knee will be closer to ninety degrees. This puts a lot of weight through the kneecap, so supporting the back knee with a bolster or rolled blanket can help.

Prop option:
- ▷ If your kneecaps or the tops of your ankles are sensitive, you can place a small cushion or blanket under them for extra cushioning.
- ▷ A bolster or rolled blanket can be placed to rest on your back hip/thigh.
- ▷ Blocks can be placed under the hands.
- ▷ A strap can be used to increase the stretch along the front of the thigh.

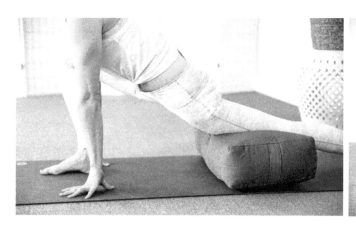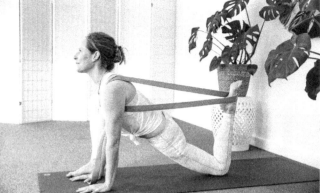

Variations:

High Dragon

▷ Lift your chest and bring your hands or forearms to rest on your front thigh or on upright blocks.

▷ This increases the stretch along the front of your torso and the front of your back, hip, and thigh.

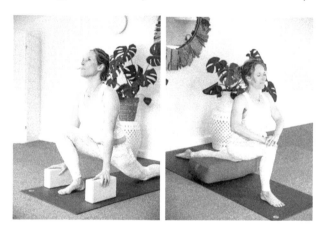

Tennis Ball Dragon

▷ Place a tennis ball or spiky ball under the front foot and gently massage your plantar fascia whilst in dragon or High Dragon. Slowly shift your weight through your front leg to allow for the foot massage.

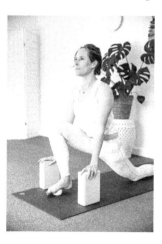

Low Winged Dragon

▷ Both hands are in front of you. You may be able to rest your forearms down onto the floor.

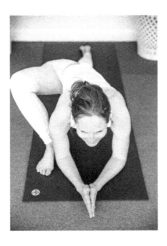

Low Winged Dragon with Twist

> ▷ From Low Dragon, allow your front knee to wing outwards.
> ▷ Use your opposite hand to push the front knee to the side to maintain its "wing" and turn your torso towards your wing and the sky.
> ▷ A deeper version of this is available, where you continue into the twist, bend your posterior (back) knee, and hold onto your dragon tail.

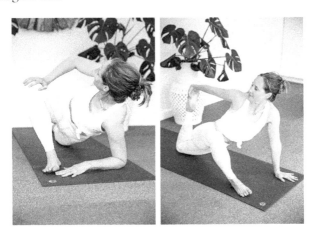

Eagle Arms / Garuda

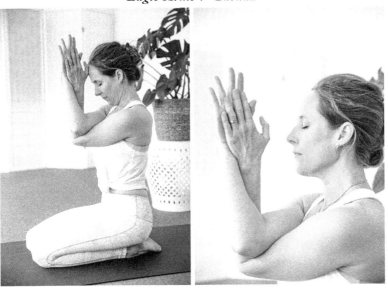

Target area:
- ▷ Stretches along the Heart, Pericardium, Triple Warmer, Lung, Small and Large Intestine meridians
- ▷ Stretches along the back of the shoulder and arms

Practising the pose:
- ▷ Find a comfortable seated position. Bring the right arm out in front, place the left elbow underneath the right elbow, bend the elbows and bring the palms together.
- ▷ If you can't bring your palms together, straighten the right arm and draw it across your torso, towards the left, using your left arm, and keep your arms low.
- ▷ A slight twist through the torso can help increase the stretch along the back of the shoulder.
- ▷ Slowly swap sides. Remember each side often feels quite different and may look very different, and that's OK.

Hold time:
- ▷ One to three minutes

Variations:

Standing or Supine Eagle Arms

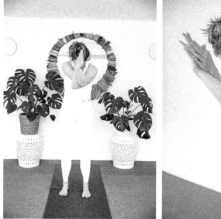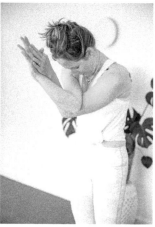

Soaring Eagle
- ▷ Allow your eagle to soar by moving your elbows up and away from your torso, arching your spine, and lifting your chin.

Eye of Needle

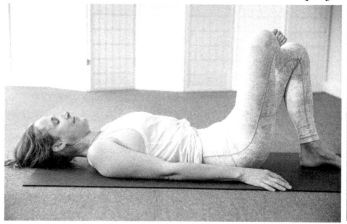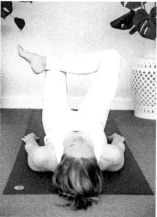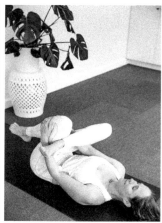

Target area:
- ▷ Stretches gluteal, piriformis, and tensor fascia lata muscles
- ▷ Externally rotates the hip on the chosen side
- ▷ Stretches the Gall Bladder meridian

Practising the pose:
- ▷ From lying on your back with both knees bent, draw your right knee in towards your chest.
- ▷ Flex your right foot (draw your right toes towards your right knee) as you cross your right foot over your body and rest your right ankle just above your left knee.
- ▷ This might be enough sensation and stretch for some.
- ▷ Once you have your right foot comfortably in position, consciously relax your feet.
- ▷ For more sensation, hug your left knee towards your chest, deepening the right external hip rotation.
- ▷ Relax your shoulders and head. Make sure they are resting on the mat and/or pillow.
- ▷ Hold. Slowly come out of the pose and swap sides.

Hold time:
- ▷ One to three minutes

Caution:
- ▷ If you have knee issues, try crossing your legs with your thighs touching and your knees closer together.

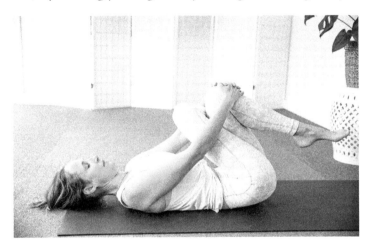

Variation:

Wall Eye of Needle
- ▷ From Wall Caterpillar bend your right knee and flex your right foot as you bring your right foot to rest above your left knee. This may be enough stretch/sensation for you.
- ▷ For more sensation, start to bend your left leg, keeping your left foot on the wall.
- ▷ Relax your feet.
- ▷ You may like to place your right hand on your right knee and gently push towards the wall to help increase external hip rotation.
- ▷ Hold. Slowly release back into Wall Caterpillar and then swap sides.

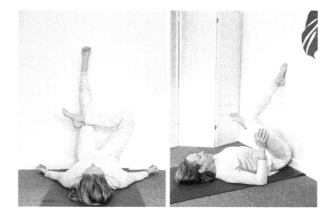

Frog

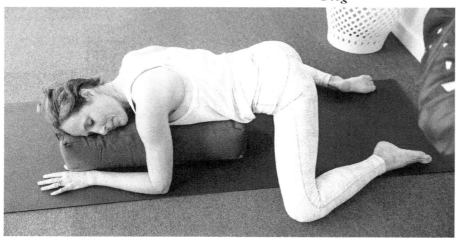
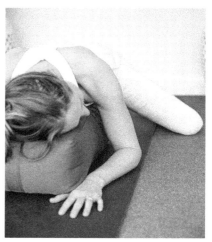

Target area:
  ▷ Stretches the inner groin and hips
  ▷ Stretches the Liver, Kidney, and Spleen meridians

Practising the pose:
  ▷ Start in a wide knee Child's Pose. Shift your weight forward and bring weight into your arms.
  ▷ Hold. Feel into the stretch through the groin and hips.
  ▷ To come out of the pose, either shift back into Child's Pose or slide forward onto your belly.

Hold time:
  ▷ Two to three minutes

Caution:
  ▷ Individual hip anatomy will impact how this pose looks for each person.
  ▷ Avoid this pose if you have low back issues.

Props:
  ▷ You may like to place extra padding under the knees.
  ▷ You may like to lie on a booster or stack of pillows. This provides extra support for your torso and can decrease the intensity of the stretch through the inner groin.

Variations:

Half Frog
- ▷ From lying on your belly, draw one leg out to the side to create a one-sided groin stretch.
- ▷ Turn your head towards the bent knee.

Happy Baby

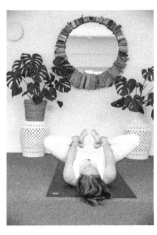 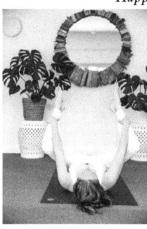 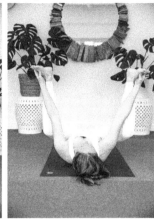 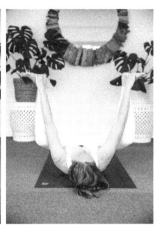

Target area:
- ▷ Deep and juicy hip stretch
- ▷ Releases and decompresses the sacroiliac joints
- ▷ Stretches the Kidney, Liver, Urinary Bladder, and Gall Bladder meridians

Practising the pose:
- ▷ From lying on your back, hug your knees up to your chest.
- ▷ Widen the knees; we are looking for a deep stretch in the hips and groin.
- ▷ You can hold onto your knees, the back of your thighs, shins, or ankles. Or you may be able to hold onto the soles of your feet.
- ▷ Relax your head and neck.
- ▷ This pose tends to get juicier the longer you hold it.
- ▷ To come out of the pose, slowly release your hold on the legs and bring your feet back onto the floor. Rebound in CRP or Savasana.

Hold time:
- ▷ Two to five minutes

Caution:
- ▷ If you have sacroiliac sprain or acute low back pain, avoid this pose.

Props:
- ▷ You may find placing a bolster or rolled blanket under the pelvis helpful.
- ▷ Placing a pillow under the head can help the head and neck relax.
- ▷ You can place a strap around the soles of the feet and hold on to it, rather than holding onto your legs/feet.

Variation:

One-Leg Happy Baby
- ▷ From lying on your back, bend and hold onto one leg/foot whilst the opposite leg is out long.

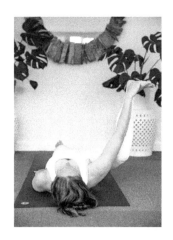

Lizard

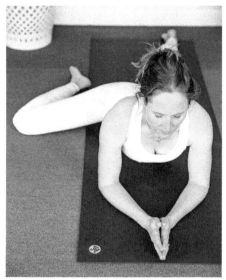 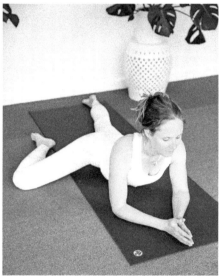 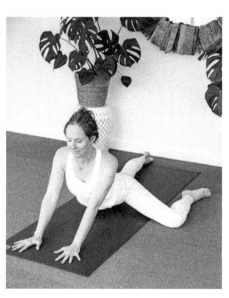

Target area:
  ▷ Stretches along the inner groin, into the hip, and along the front of the torso
  ▷ Stretches the Spleen, Stomach, Liver, Kidney, and Gall Bladder meridians

Practising the pose:
  ▷ From lying on your belly, bend and draw your right leg out to the side to a ninety-degree angle.
  ▷ Come up onto your elbows, like in sphinx pose. (If this is too uncomfortable, stay in Half Frog, with only the leg out to the side and no arm involvement.)
  ▷ To increase sensation further, you can straighten your arms like in seal pose.
  ▷ Hold. Feel into the groin and hip on the bent leg side.
  ▷ To come out of the pose, release the arms first, bring your torso back to the mat, and then release your leg so both legs are out long.
  ▷ Prone rebound before swapping sides.

Hold time:
  ▷ One to three minutes

Caution:
  ▷ If you have a sacroiliac sprain, avoid this pose.
  ▷ Low back pain.

Melting Heart / Anahatasana

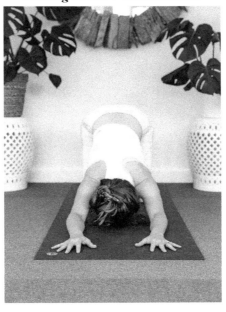

Target area:
- ▷ Stretches along the arms, shoulders, and front of the chest/torso
- ▷ Stretches the Lung, Pericardium and Heart meridians running along the arms

Practising the pose:
- ▷ From all fours, walk your arms forward.
- ▷ Keep your hips aligned above your knees and melt your heart towards the floor.
- ▷ Allow your back to arch/extend.
- ▷ This pose can be too intense for some. Try Half Melting Heart and/or bolster under the chest.
- ▷ Hold. Allow your heart to melt a little further towards the floor with each exhalation.
- ▷ Slowly come out of the pose by pushing back to all fours on an inhalation.
- ▷ Rebound in Child's Pose or Prone Rebound.

Hold time:
- ▷ Two to five minutes

Caution:
- ▷ Be careful if you have any shoulder or neck issues. You do not want to feel any shoulder compression.
- ▷ This pose can be too strong for some people. Try Half Melting Heart instead.

Props:
- ▷ You may like a bolster under the chest, under the forearms, or under the knees; try which suits you best.

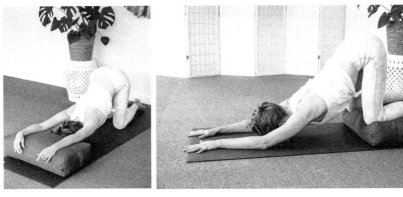

Variation:

Half Melting Heart

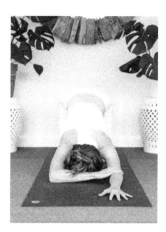

> ▷ Only one arm is out long. The other is bent, and you can rest your forehead on your bent forearm.
> ▷ This option is less intense.
> ▷ Swap sides halfway through the time that has been allowed for Melting Heart.

Saddle

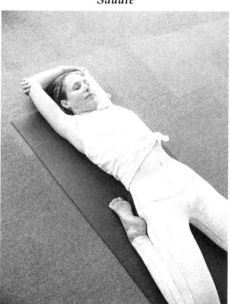

Target area:
> ▷ Stretches along the front of the thighs, hips, and torso
> ▷ Stretches hip flexors and quadriceps
> ▷ Stretches along the Stomach, Spleen, and Kidney meridians
> ▷ Compresses the Urinary Bladder meridians

Practising the pose:
> ▷ Start with sitting on your heels, knees bent. (If this is already painful, avoid this pose.)
> ▷ Lean back on your hands, this might already be enough of a stretch for you, so hold here.
> ▷ You can increase sensation by leaning back onto your elbows, creating an arch/extension in the spine. Some people can come all the way down and rest their torso on the floor.
> ▷ Slowly and carefully come out of this pose. It can be easiest to roll towards one side to gently come out. Rebound in CRP or Savasana.

Hold time:
- ▷ One to five minutes

Caution:
- ▷ Avoid this pose if you have a sacroiliac sprain.
- ▷ Avoid this pose if you have current low back pain.
- ▷ Can be too much for some ankles and knees. Try half saddle or using props or avoid.
- ▷ Supported Saddle and Half Saddle are gentler versions.

Variations:

Supported Saddle

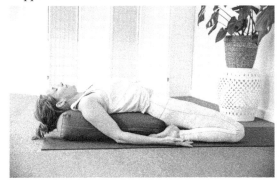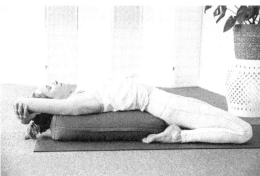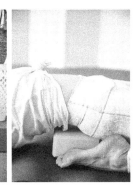

Half Saddle
- ▷ One leg is bent whilst one leg stays out long.
- ▷ Do not force the pelvis to be level (individual hip anatomy will result in the pose looking different for each of us, yet we will still feel into the same target area).
- ▷ A side-lying Half Saddle can help some people access the same stretch without so much pressure on the front of the ankles and knees. A strap can also be used in a side-lying Half Saddle to relieve any arm discomfort or tension.

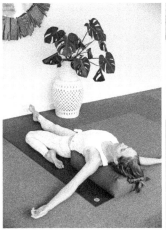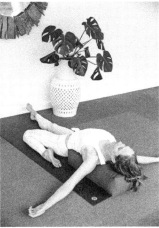

Sphinx

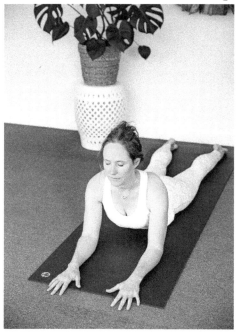 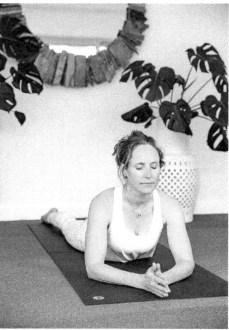

Target area:
  ▷ Stretches along the front of the torso
  ▷ Compresses/squashes the lower back
  ▷ Stretches along the Kidney, Stomach, Spleen, and Liver meridians.
  ▷ Urinary Bladder and Kidney meridians are compressed where they run through the lower back and sacrum

Practising the pose:
  ▷ From lying on your belly, gently come up on to your elbows into a backbend.
  ▷ Make sure your elbows are aligned a little farther forward of your shoulders. You might like your palms face down or in a prayer position.
  ▷ Take a few moments to find your Goldilocks position; elbows wide will decrease sensation in your lower back, elbows closer together will increase sensation in your lower back. You might like to have legs close together or a little apart.
  ▷ Feel into the target areas—a squashed sensation in your lower back and a stretch along the front of the torso.
  ▷ If sensation is too much in your lower back, try Lizard Pose (swap sides halfway through the time allocated for sphinx) or rest in Prone Rebound.
  ▷ To come out of the pose slowly release on an exhalation into prone rebound.
  ▷ Note, it is normal to initially feel a little fragile in the target area of the low back when we rebound out of Sphinx.

Hold time:
  ▷ Two to five minutes.

Caution:
  ▷ Low back pain.
  ▷ Some people with a lumbar disc bulge or herniation find this pose very therapeutic.
  ▷ If pregnant, rest your pelvis up on a side-positioned bolster or a stack of pillows. This pose can create delicious space for the belly and torso.

Prop options:

▷ A bolster or rolled blanket can be placed under the ribcage, under the bra line. This can take pressure off the neck and shoulders.

▷ A blanket or pillow under the pelvis can remove pubic discomfort.

▷ You can cup the chin with your hands to support your head and neck.

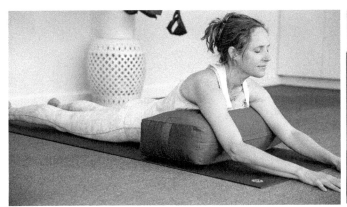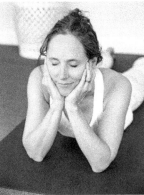

Variations:

Wall Sphinx

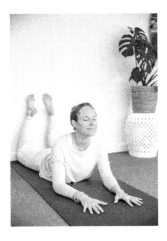

▷ Rest the tops of your feet against the wall with your knees bent in Sphinx. Wall Sphinx is a stronger version of Sphinx.

Seal

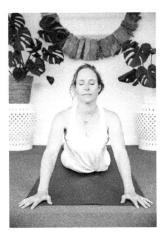

▷ From Sphinx, gently straighten the arms to increase sensation in the low back. Place your palms mat-width apart.

▷ To further increase sensation, you can walk the palms closer to your pelvis.

Square

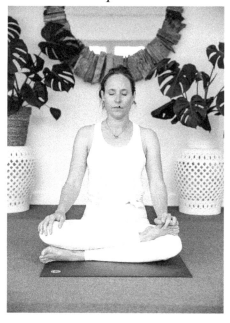

Target area:
    ▷ Deeply stretches the hips through external rotation
    ▷ Stretches the Liver, Kidney, and Gall Bladder meridians
    ▷ Stretches the Urinary Bladder meridians when folded forward
    ▷ Stretches the Heart and Small Intestine meridians with side stretch
    ▷ Twists through the spine and Spleen, Stomach, Kidney, and Liver meridians with added twist.

Practising the pose:
    ▷ Start in a seated position with your legs crossed. Bring your right foot to rest on top of your left knee. Your left foot rests under your right knee, and your shins stack on top of each other. If this is too intense, place the right foot on the ground just in front of the left knee.
    ▷ Gently fold forward to increase sensation.
    ▷ Hold. Feel into the hips. Some people will feel a lower back stretch too.
    ▷ Slowly come out of the pose into Seated Rebound and/or Windscreen Wipers before swapping sides.

Note: Some people with a lumbar disc bulge or herniation find this pose very therapeutic.

Hold time:
    ▷ Two to five minutes

Caution:
    ▷ Avoid this pose if it results in knee pain. An alternative pose is eye of needle.
    ▷ Keep an upright spine position if your neck or low back are feeling vulnerable.
    ▷ This pose can aggravate sciatica. Placing a pillow or folded blanket under the pelvis can help.

Prop options:
    ▷ You may like to support the knees with blocks or a rolled blanket.
    ▷ A pillow or folded blanket under the pelvis will tilt the pelvis forward.

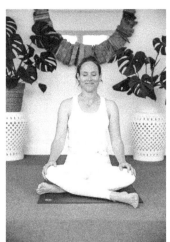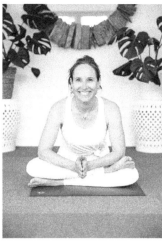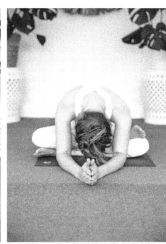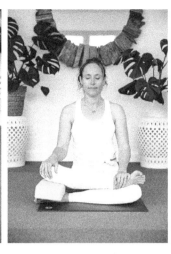

Variation:

Square Pose with Side Stretch
> ▷ Whilst in upright square, you can bring an arm up over head and lean to the opposite side, causing a stretch along the side body. You can rest the lower elbow on the floor or on top of a block or bolster and support your head with this lower hand.
> ▷ Hold. Feel into the opening along the side of the torso, shoulder, and arm.
> ▷ Gently come out of the pose on an inhalation, swap square pose side, and then repeat with opposite arm above.

Supported Bridge

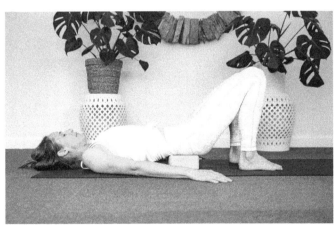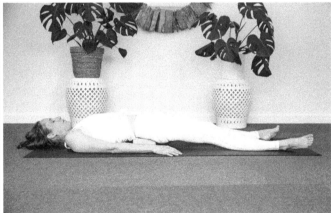

Target area:
> ▷ Stretches along the front of the torso and arches/extends the lower back.
> ▷ Stretches the Stomach, Spleen, Kidney, Urinary Bladder, and Liver meridians.
> ▷ With arms overhead Lung, Pericardium and Heart meridians are stretched.

Practising the pose:
> ▷ From lying on your back, bend your knees and bring your heels in close to your buttocks.
> ▷ Gently lift your pelvis on your inhalation and place a yoga block or thick hardcover book underneath your pelvis. Place it underneath your sacrum, *not* under your lower lumbar spine.
> ▷ You may like to place two blocks underneath your sacrum if it feels comfortable to increase the stretch along the front of your hips and torso.

▷ Next, choose your leg placement; both legs can remain bent, or both legs can be stretched out long.

▷ You can keep your arms by your side or bring both up to rest on the floor above your head to increase sensation.

▷ Hold. Feel into your torso, front of hips, and arms if overhead. This is a gentle inversion.

▷ To come out of the pose, breathe in and lift your pelvis up to gently remove the block. As you breathe out, slowly return your pelvis and spine back to the mat, rolling back down vertebrae by vertebrae. Your sacrum is the last spinal bone to meet the mat.

▷ Pause and rebound in CRP. Feel the support of the ground underneath you. It is normal to feel a little achy in the lower back whilst we rebound out of Supported Bridge.

Hold time:

▷ Three to five minutes

Caution:

▷ Take care if you currently have low back pain, arthritic hips, reflux, abdominal hernia, eye issues or recent surgery.

▷ This pose is contraindicated in people with anterolisthesis and anterior total hip replacement.

▷ Avoid if pregnant. Do Sphinx or Seal with pelvic support instead.

Prop options:

▷ If the yoga block feels too hard/uncomfortable, you may like to use a bolster or supportive pillow placed under the pelvis instead.

▷ If your spine is feeling vulnerable, you can take most of it out of the equation by lying on a bolster or pile of blankets lengthwise, with your torso and head supported.

Variation:

One-Leg Supported Bridge

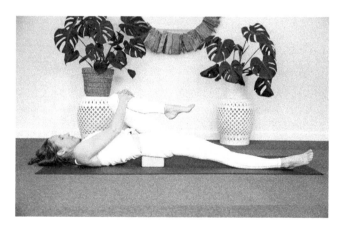

▷ From Supported Bridge with both knees bent, gently straighten the right leg. Feel for a stretch along the front of the right hip.

▷ You can hug your left knee into your chest to increase sensation if required.

▷ To come out of the pose slowly release the hug of the left knee and place the left foot back on the floor; bend your right knee to meet your left.

▷ Rebound for a few moments, resting with your pelvis evenly placed on the block before swapping sides.

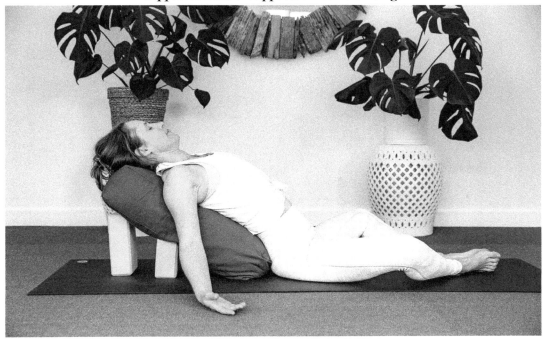

Target area:
- ▷ Stretches across the front of the chest and torso
- ▷ Stretches along the arms
- ▷ Stretches the Kidney, Spleen, Stomach, Heart, Pericardium, and Lung meridians

Practising the pose:
- ▷ Set two blocks up with a bolster or large pillow resting on top (like in the photo). You can also just use blocks, but this will make it hard to transition into Lounging Monkey.
- ▷ Gently recline back to allow a stretch across the front of your chest and down your arms.
- ▷ There are various options for your legs—crossed legs, soles of feet together in Butterfly, legs straight, or legs bent with knees together like in CRP.
- ▷ You can progress deeper into the pose by moving into Lounging Monkey
- ▷ To come out of the pose gently roll off to one side, come off your props, and rest in Side-lying Rebound.

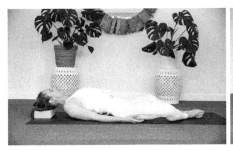 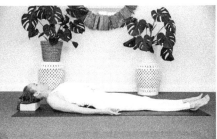 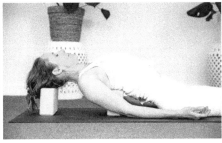

Hold time:
- ▷ Three to five minutes

Caution:
- ▷ Be extra careful getting in and out of the pose if you have a sensitive low back. You may like to gently roll over to one side to come out of the pose.

Supported Lounging Monkey

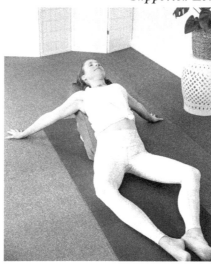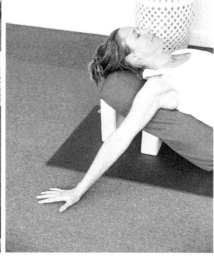

Target area:
- ▷ Stretches across the front of the chest and torso
- ▷ Stretches along the arms
- ▷ Stretches the Kidney, Spleen, Stomach, Lung, Heart, Pericardium, and Small Intestine meridians.

Practising the pose:
- ▷ From Supported Thoracic Bridge, slowly finger walk your arms farther back behind you to increase the stretch through the front of the chest, shoulders, and arms (be careful of shoulder compression).

Hold time:
- ▷ Two to three minutes

Caution:
- ▷ This is quite a strong pose. You do not want to feel any shoulder or neck compression. Be careful with your arm placement.
- ▷ Avoid if you have a history of recurrent shoulder dislocations.

Toe Stretch

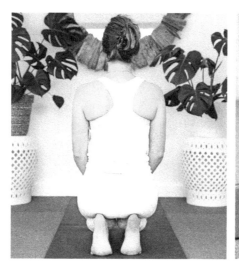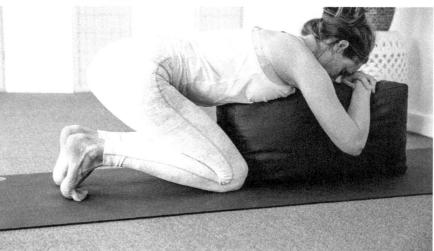

Target area:
- ▷ Strong stretch through the plantar fascia (connective tissue of the feet) which stimulates all the lower body meridians-Stomach, Spleen, Liver, Gall Bladder, Kidney and Urinary Bladder.

Practising the pose:

  ▷ Lean forward from child's pose and tuck your toes under. You might like to position your feet and knees together or slightly apart.

  ▷ Make sure all your toes are tucked, including your little toes. You may have to use your hands to help get your toes into place.

  ▷ This can be a very intense stretch along the soles of the feet and toes, along your plantar fascia. Have a little play with shifting your body weight forwards and backwards to help find your Goldilocks position. You can decrease the stretch by shifting your body weight forwards and even rest your torso over a bolster or increase the stretch by sitting upright over the toes.

  ▷ Slowly come out of the pose by leaning forwards and releasing your toes; give them a gentle shake or roll. You might like to move into Ankle Stretch from here.

Hold time:

  ▷ Thirty seconds to three minutes (depending on tolerance)

Caution:

  ▷ Take care if you have knee issues and/or ankle issues.

  ▷ Avoid or attempt very carefully if you have past ankle and toe fractures.

Variations:

  ▷ If you're able to sit upright over the toes, you can add an arm and thoracic stretch with Garuda Arms or slow finger stretches.

Twists

Target area:

  ▷ Gentle twist through the spine and opening up of one side of the chest at a time

  ▷ Stretches and squeezes the Gall Bladder and Urinary Bladder meridians

  ▷ Squeezes the Spleen, Stomach, Kidney, and Liver meridians

  ▷ The twist through the torso gently squeezes the abdominal organs, which helps the body digest any food and/or any emotions that arise during practice

  ▷ When arms are placed in a cactus arm position or out ninety degrees this stimulates all the upper body meridians—Heart, Lung, Small and Large Intestine, Triple Warmer, and Pericardium.

Hold time:

  ▷ Three to five minutes

Caution:

  ▷ Cactus arm position can be too strong if you have any shoulder issues. Keep arms in a low angel wings position instead (see photos).

Variations:

One-Leg Twist

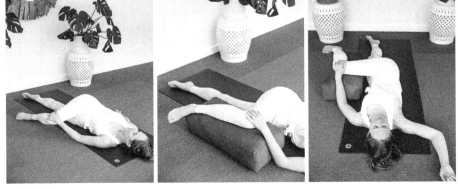

Practising the pose:

▷ From lying on your back with your legs long, bend your right knee and hug it to your chest.

▷ Twist your body to the left, whilst drawing your right knee across your torso.

▷ You may like to rest your right knee on a block or bolster for support.

▷ Hold your right knee with your left hand.

▷ Place your right arm in a low angel wing position.

▷ Hold. Feel into the twist and breathe down into your belly.

▷ Slowly roll out of the pose and bring your pelvis back to the centre of the mat.

▷ Rebound in CRP or Savasana before swapping sides.

Reclining Twist

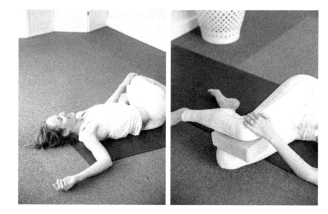

Practising the pose:

▷ Place both feet on the floor with your heels close to your buttocks. Inhale and lift your pelvis up. Shift it across to the right side of your mat. As you exhale, drop your pelvis back onto the floor and let your bent knees drop over to the left side.

▷ You may like to place a block/bolster under or between the knees for support.

▷ You may like your right arm to stay in a low angel wing, or come out ninety degrees to your side, or come up into a cactus arm position.

▷ Find a comfortable position for your head, facing forwards or resting to left or right.

▷ Hold. Feel the twist through the spine and the opening of the right side of the chest. Belly breathe.

▷ To come out of the pose, slowly draw your arms down alongside your torso on an exhalation and then bring your knees back upright, uncross them, and rebound in CRP or Savasana.

Twisted Roots

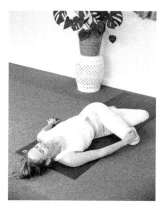

Practising the pose:

▷ This pose is similar to Reclining Twist but cross your legs at the start; cross your right leg over the top of your left before you lift and shift your pelvis to the right side of your mat on inhalation. As you exhale, allow your crossed legs to drop to the left side of the mat.

▷ You may like to place a block/bolster under the knees for support.

▷ Next choose your arm position. You may like your right arm to stay in a low angel wing or bring it out to the side ninety degrees or bring it up into a cactus arm position.

▷ Find a comfortable position for your head, facing forwards or resting to left or right.

▷ Hold. Feel the twist through the spine and the opening of the right side of the chest. Belly breathe.

▷ To come out of the pose, slowly draw your arms down alongside your torso on an exhalation and then bring your knees back upright and uncross them.

▷ Rebound in CRP or Savasana and then swap sides.

Seated Twist

Practising the pose:

▷ From a seated position, Square or Butterfly, cross your legs with your right leg on top.

▷ Hold onto your right knee or thigh, inhale and lift through the chest, and exhale and twist to look over your right shoulder.

▷ Place your right hand behind you for support.

▷ Hold. Feel the twist through the spine and the opening of the right side of the chest.

▷ To come out of the pose, slowly release your twist and return to face forwards. Rebound in Seated Rebound, or you may prefer some yang Windscreen Wipers before you swap sides.

Wall Squat

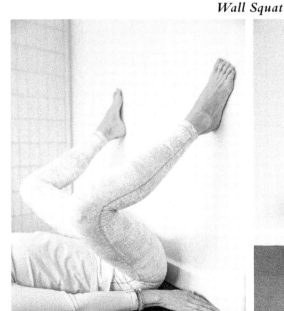 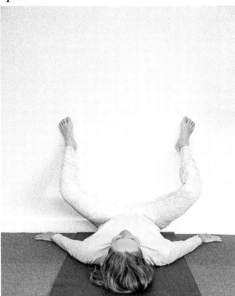

Target area:

▷ Deeply stretches hips and groin

▷ Stretches Gall Bladder, Liver, and Kidney meridians

Practising the pose:

▷ From wall caterpillar bend your knees, keep the soles of your feet on the wall, and slide your feet out and downwards until you reach a squat position.

▷ Play with your feet position on the wall until you find your Goldilocks position, feeling sensation deep in your hips.

▷ This pose helps open the hips and can offer relief from low back pain associated with your period.

▷ Slowly come out of the pose by hugging your knees to your chest or move into Wall Caterpillar.

Hold time:
  ▷ Three to five minutes

Caution:
  ▷ If hips are really tight, this can torque the knees and strain them. Play with the position of your feet on the wall so your knees feel comfortable.

Wings

Hold time:
  ▷ One to three minutes (Arm poses can be more intense. Please modify or come out of the pose if you notice any tingles or "zinging" in the arms.)

Embracing Wings / Closed Wings

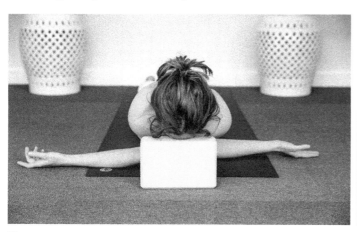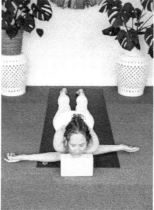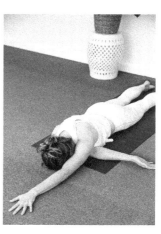

Target area:
  ▷ Stretches along the back of the arm and shoulder
  ▷ Stretches along the Triple Warmer, Small and Large Intestine meridians.

Practising the pose:
  ▷ From lying on your belly, prop yourself up on your elbows temporarily to thread your right arm through, landing your right shoulder and arm on the mat. We are looking for a stretch along the back of the right arm and shoulder.
  ▷ You can choose to embrace one wing/arm at a time or both (see photo variations).
  ▷ Next, tuck your toes under to push your torso up towards the top of your mat. This can increase the stretch along the back of your arm, and it can help relieve pressure on breast tissue.
  ▷ You can vary the position of your legs to increase or decrease the stretch. You can keep legs long or try a Half Frog leg position on either side to find which suits you best.
  ▷ Hold. Belly breathe.
  ▷ Slowly move into Prone Rebound and pause for one minute before you swap sides.

Prop options:
  ▷ You may like to use a block to support the head with chin up or down.
  ▷ You may like a blanket or pillow positioned under the breast line to relieve pressure/compression of your breasts.

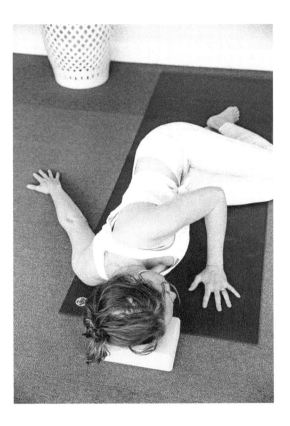

Target area:
- ▷ Stretches along the front of the shoulder and chest. You may feel the stretch along the arm too.
- ▷ Stretches along the Heart, Pericardium, and Lung meridians.

Practising the pose:
- ▷ From lying on your side, draw your right arm behind you forty-five to ninety degrees, with your palm facing up or down.
- ▷ Use a block or pillow for head support if helpful.
- ▷ Leg position and props impact sensation in the arms. See various options in photos below.
- ▷ Some people can come into double Open Wings (see photo).

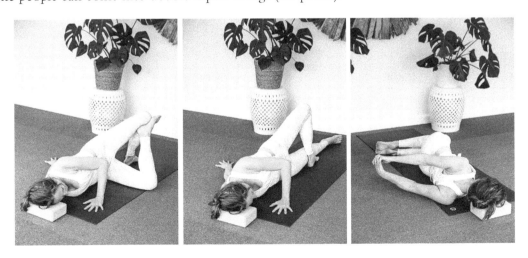

Yang Asanas

Cat/Cow

▷ Start on all fours. Have your hips lined up above your knees and your shoulders in line with your hands.

▷ You can place your palms down on the floor, or you can come up onto fingertips and thumb tips if you have the hand strength, or you can rest on your knuckles with a closed fist with your thumbs out pressing down on the mat. Your hand position and direction of pressure placed through your fingers and/or thumbs can impact different meridian end points and start points; thumbs – LU11, index fingers – LI1, middle fingers – PC9, ring fingers – TH1, little fingers – HT9 and SI1. Further clarification can be found on the individual meridian diagrams found in each seasonal practice found in Part II.

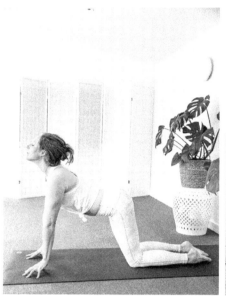 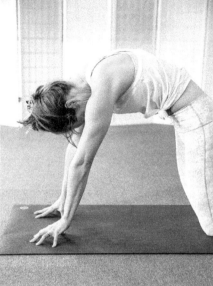 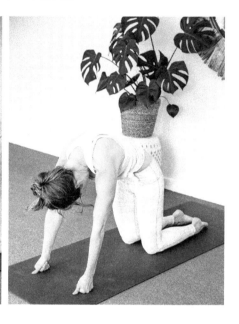

Knee Squeeze Roll Back

▷ From a seated position, with legs out in front of you, place a block between your bent knees.

▷ If your core is feeling strong, hold your arms out in front of you with your palms facing upwards.

▷ If your core is feeling tired or weak, hold onto your knees.

▷ Breathe in, squeeze the block between bent knees and lift up through the torso. Activate your pelvic floor, your mula bandha, and your core abdominal muscles.

▷ Breathe out, squeeze the block between bent knees, and keep your core activated as you slowly roll back vertebrae by vertebrae until you are lying down on the mat.

Pelvic Tilts

▷ Lie on your back, bend your knees, and bring your heels to rest on the floor close to your buttocks.

▷ Breathe in, lift your pelvis up towards the sky and squeeze your buttock/gluteal muscles.

▷ Breathe out, slowly curl your spine back down onto the mat. Your sacrum, the large triangular bone at the base of your spine, should be the last bone to touch the mat.

▷ Repeat for another two or five rounds.

Knees to Chest

▷ Lying on your back, hug your knees into your chest and gently massage your low back by slowly rocking side to side.

Windscreen Wipers

▷ Whilst seated, place your palms down behind you and lean back onto your hands.
▷ Loosely bend your knees, with your knees wide apart, and slowly drop your knees from one side to the other. This moves your hips through internal and external rotation.

Rebound Asanas

As you rest in stillness in the rebound asanas, please draw attention towards your body sensations and your breath. As you increase your inner awareness, your inner seeing and listening, you are increasing your interoception and ability to access your intuition.

Constructive Rest Pose (CRP)

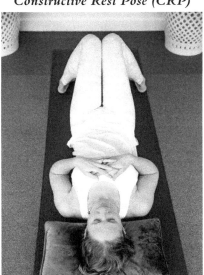

▷ Lying on your back, bend your knees.
▷ With your feet apart resting on the floor, let your knees knock together.

Prone Rebound

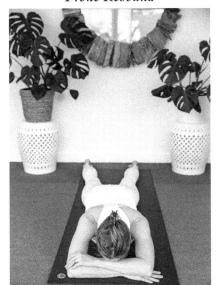

▷ Lying on your belly, rest your head on your stacked forearms.

▷ As you inhale, feel your belly pressing against the mat. As you exhale, relax, and let go.

Savasana / Supine Rebound

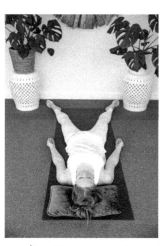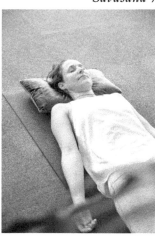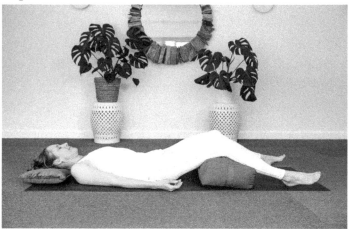

▷ Lie on your back, legs slightly apart, palms open resting by your side or on your belly.

▷ You may like to slightly bend the knees and place a pillow underneath them for support to take a little pressure off your lower back.

Seated Anjali Mudra

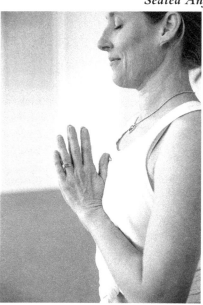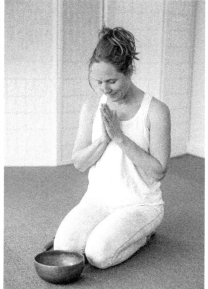

▷ Come into a comfortable seated position, bring your palms in prayer in front of your heart, and gently bow your head.

▷ When we finish our practice, we can bring our thumbs to your third eye centre as a gesture of honour, respect, and gratitude.

Seated Rebound

▷ From an upright seated position, place your palms behind you, lean back onto straight arms, and straighten your legs out in front.

▷ Lift your chest and open your heart to the sky.

Side-Lying Rebound

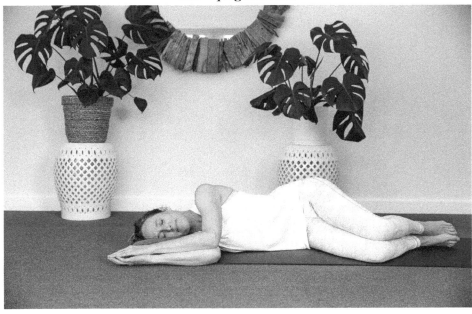

▷ Lie on your side with your knees bent and stacked on top of each other and elbows bent and stacked on top of each other.

Third Eye Centre / Anja

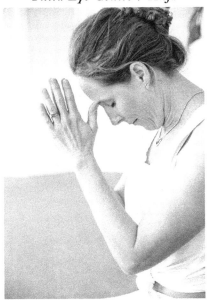

▷ Located in the centre of your forehead, in line with the middle of your eyebrows.
▷ Is believed to be linked to perception, awareness, and spiritual communication.

Chapter 7
Meditate with the Seasons

Meditation

There are many inspiring and informative books on meditation already out in the world, so we will not be delving deep here. Instead, I share with you an introduction to meditation, finding your "why," some seasonal meditation insights, and some of the practices I teach (these go alongside the gratitude and compassion practices I have shared earlier).

I am so fortunate to have had the meditation teachers I've had. Bob Sharples is one of my teachers, and he is very dear to my heart. His introduction to meditation, in *Meditation: Calming the Mind*, is gentle and insightful: "Don't meditate to fix yourself, to improve yourself, to redeem yourself; rather, do it as an act of love, of deep warm friendship to yourself. In this way there is no longer any need for the subtle aggression of self-improvement, for the endless guilt of not doing enough. It offers the possibility of an end to the ceaseless round of trying so hard that wraps so many people's lives in a knot. Instead, there is now meditation as an act of love. How endlessly delightful and encouraging."[1]

The word *meditation* comes from the Latin word *meditari*. Medatari means frequent. So, we know we are to practise frequently. Yet there is nothing in the word to explain what it is we actually do. This imprecision of the word is actually quite useful. It allows you to choose which method/technique suits you best. I share a few different meditation practices in this book. Please choose which one(s) resonate with you.

Meditation is not:
- Tuning out and having an outer body experience
- About achieving, accomplishing, conquering, or succeeding
- About planning, solving, worrying, helping, or thinking
- A religion, cult, or fad

Meditation is both an ancient science and an art form. There are fundamental techniques and skills you learn to apply in a systematic and structured manner. Just as we train our muscles for strength and stability, we can use meditation techniques and skills to help train our attention and awareness. We can train our mind. And just like creating art, with regular practice you will improve and be able to find your own style.

Bob has shared many wonderful and enlightening poems with me over the years. I have him to thank for my love of poetry—hence the poems dotted throughout this book. I find that poetry communicates with and caresses our inner awareness, our aware mind. He introduced me to the wonderful works of current female poet Kaveri Patel. Her poetry resonates deeply with me, and she has graciously and generously allowed me to share some of her works with you in this book. My hope is that you may find her poems helpful too. Here is a poem she has written on meditation:

"A New and Deeper Truth"
(from Under the Waves)

the old truth made you
run a thousand miles
inside an arid desert
desperate for an oasis

sit and close your eyes
inhale the breeze of kindness
exhale the toxic judgments
dehydrating you like a prune

feel the pain of old patterns
trapped in tense muscles
it's ok to cry, to taste
the salt of possibility

just be, just breathe
let waves break against
the silence, returning you
to a new and deeper truth[2]

You can listen to Kaveri recite this poem on her website, Wisdom in Waves, found at https://www.wisdominwaves.com/about.html.

Meditation teaches us how to breathe and be with the truth of each moment, whether it is pleasant or unpleasant. It takes courage to be with things as they are. As we practise regularly, with patience and an open heart, we gain perspective and discernment. We can begin to observe our active "monkey mind" and notice and then understand its tendencies and cheeky patterns of negativity. Daily meditation practice allows for discovery.

Meditation helps us develop patience, kindness, and a sense of humour. It offers us the opportunity to reconnect with ourselves and, over time, to develop an unconditional friendship with ourselves. Meditation allows us to be open and receptive to the whisperings and insight of our body. It allows us to develop our intuition and wonder.

Why meditate?

If you are just beginning your journey with meditation, or even if you have a well-established practice, it is helpful to know *why* you are meditating. Mindfulness meditation is simple but not always easy. There will be days when you just don't feel like it, or you might feel like you don't have the time. The first six to eight weeks are usually the hardest when trying to make daily meditation a new habit. So, working out *why* you are meditating in the first place will help you stay on the path and hold the thread. Your why may change along the way, and that's OK.

The following list of benefits of mindfulness meditation, courtesy of the Living Valley Centre, was shared during the mindfulness-based stillness meditation (MBSM) teacher training I attended there. See if you can find one or more reasons as to why *you* want to meditate:

The Wonderful Benefits of Meditation

1. It relaxes the body and calms the mind.
2. It reduces stress and anxiety.
3. It helps you connect to yourself, to others, and to the natural world.
4. It increases self-awareness, self-acceptance, and self-compassion.
5. It helps decrease judgement of others and of yourself.
6. It increases perspective.
7. It helps develop kindness, empathy, compassion, and courage.
8. It helps you learn to distinguish between yourself and your thoughts. Everything changes; thoughts come and go, nothing is permanent.
9. It increases resilience; you become less disturbed by and less reactive to unpleasant experiences and emotions.
10. It helps you safely experience uncomfortable thoughts and emotions.
11. It decreases emotional reactivity.
12. It helps develop your ability to listen deeply and speak your truth.
13. It helps to lighten things up and helps you be less burdened by seriousness and over-responsibility.
14. It helps develop the ability to stay grounded, centred, and composed, even amid turmoil.
15. It improves mental clarity, concentration, memory, and cognition.
16. It improves relaxation.
17. It balances blood pressure and immune function.
18. It improves energy levels and reduces fatigue.

Seasonal Resistance

Forms of resistance occur during meditation and a slow asana practice like yin yoga. They are normal and to be expected. They are withdrawal symptoms from stimulus addiction, worrying, planning, and constant doing.

Resistance forms:

- Boredom
- Sleepiness/drowsiness (this is different to exhaustion from not enough sleep)
- Restlessness
- Frustration/impatience/agitation/crankiness
- Doubt (of self, teacher, and/or the process)
- Pain

I have noticed, through teaching and my own practice, that the seasons impact these forms of resistance. During the yin seasons of autumn and winter, sleepiness and drowsiness are more frequent. Sleepiness can also commonly arise whilst practising Mindfulness of Emotions. It can help to sit to meditate during these seasons, as then there is less chance of falling asleep and/or falling into a trance-like state.

The long, achy holds of yin yoga can activate boredom, frustration, irritability, and even anger at any time of the year. But during the yang seasons of spring, summer, and late summer, these forms of resistance increase and become more intrusive. The same applies to our quiet mindful meditation practice—boredom, restlessness, agitation, impatience, procrastination, and pain arise more commonly during the yang seasons. It can help to add a little more yang-like movement into our asana practice, to help us feel more settled prior to our meditation during the yang seasons.

Knowing these patterns of resistance are normal and common can help. We can learn to recognise resistance as it arises and let it go, release it, without getting caught up in its story. The key is to notice any forms of resistance yet persevere with the practice.

Meditation Practices

Within you there is a stillness and sanctuary to which you can retreat at any time and be yourself.

—Herman Hesse.

The following order of meditation practices was shared with me by Paul Bedson, whilst I was undergoing my meditation teacher training at the Yarra Valley Living Centre. He has generously agreed to allow me to share them with you in this book. Each practice builds on the previous, eventually bringing us to the full MBSM practice. You can practise any of these guided meditations at any time, though, and you will find my recordings of them on Insight Timer.

Mindfulness of Breath Practice

Take a few moments to find a comfortable position. If you're sitting, sit open and upright, still and strong, like a mountain.

Or if you're lying down, lie balanced and symmetrical. You may like to bend and support your knees to take pressure off your lower back.

Relax your shoulders.

Palms are open wherever they are resting.

I invite you to take a wide face-stretching yawn, with an audible release on your exhalation.

Allow all the muscles of the face to soften and your eyelids to gently close.

Draw your shoulder blades in and down your spine. Open your heart space.

You might like to take a few slow, deep belly breaths.

As you breathe out, feel your muscles softening and relaxing. Relax and let go that little bit more with each exhalation.

Ring.

Relaxing, awake and alert.

Remember there is nothing you need to be doing right now. There is nothing you need to experience or achieve during this Mindfulness of Breath Practice. This is your time.

Just let your breath settle now. Let your breath breathe you.

I invite you now to bring your attention to the *space in front of your eyes*. It's like a field of darkness. Perhaps there are some muted shapes or colours there, but we're not looking for anything. We are simply resting our attention here, in this space, with relaxed eyes and a soft gaze.

I invite you now to bring your attention to any *sounds* coming to you from outside the room. Just listen, with a gentle curiosity.

Allow the sounds to come and go without resistance.

Now bring your awareness to sounds inside the room—just listening, without judgement. Perhaps you can notice the sound of your own breath, your digestion, even your heart beating.

Allow the sounds to call your attention into the present moment—just listening.

I invite you now to draw your attention further to your *breath*. Begin to notice any sensations associated with your breath.

Notice the feeling of your breath … as you breathe in …and as you breathe out.

Feel the slight movement of your chest and your belly, rising with your in breath and falling with your out breath.

Feel the flow of air moving past your nostrils, cool on your in breath and warm on your out breath.

Just your natural breath.

Notice the slight pause between inhalation and exhalation … and the pause between exhalation and inhalation. Follow each breath.

Let your breath breathe you. You don't have to do anything.

As you notice your breath settling, know that it calms your body, heart, and mind with it, calming and releasing all through your body.

You might find it helpful to silently name your inhalation and exhalation. "Breathing in... breathing out".

If you notice your attention wandering or becoming caught up in a stream of thought, that's OK. That's what the mind does.★ Each time you notice yourself being distracted by thoughts, very gently and kindly bring your attention back to your breath. Simply notice the sensations associated with your breath. Notice any sounds. And rest your attention in the space in front of your eyes.

(Long pause.)

Ring.

As we come towards the end of this meditation, you might like to dedicate its value and virtue and send some kind thoughts.

As we breathe in, say silently to yourself, *May I be peaceful and at ease.* As we breathe out, *May others be peaceful and at ease.* As you breathe in, allow your heart to fill with that intention, and as you breathe out, send that intention out to a group or an individual.

Breathing in, *May I be peaceful and at ease.*

Breathing out, *May others be peaceful and at ease.*

Ring.

Gently start to reactive and re-energise your body now, perhaps with a wiggle of the fingers and toes, a deeper breath or two. You might like to have a stretch or give yourself a hug.

And when you're ready, you can open your eyes.

Thank you.

★No thought is a problem; no thought is important. Worrying about your thoughts is making them heavy and important. It is having thoughts about your thoughts!

Mindfulness of Body Practice

Take a moment to find a comfortable position.

If you're sitting, sit open and upright.

Or if you're lying down, lie balanced and symmetrical, legs out long. Or you may like to bend and support your knees to take pressure off your lower back.

Relax your shoulders; bring your shoulder blades down and away from your ears.

Palms are open wherever they are resting.

Your mouth is closed, soften your jaw.

I invite you to take three deep belly breaths.

As you breathe out, allow your body to soften and relax. Let go that little bit more with each exhalation.

Relaxing, awake and alert.

Remember there is nothing you need to be doing right now. There is nothing you need to accomplish or achieve during this Mindfulness of Body Practice. This is your time.

Ring.

Just let your breath settle now; let your breath breathe you.

I invite you now to bring your attention to the *space in front of your eyes.* It's like a field of darkness. Perhaps there are some muted shapes or colours there, but we're not looking for anything. Simply rest your attention here, in this space, with relaxed eyes and a soft gaze.

I invite you now to bring your attention to any *sounds* coming from outside the room. Just listen, with a gentle curiosity.

Allow the sounds to come and go without resistance. No need to judge them.

Now bring your attention to sounds inside the room, again, just listening with a gentle curiosity. Perhaps you can notice the sound of your own breath, your digestion, even your heartbeat.

Allow the sounds to call you into the present moment, just listening.

I invite you to draw your attention further to your *breath*. Notice any sensations associated with your breath.

Feel the slight movement of your chest and your belly, rising with the in breath, falling with the out breath.

Feel the flow of air moving past your nostrils, cool on the in breath and warm on the out breath.

Just let your breath breathe you; follow each breath.

Allow your breath to help anchor you into the present moment.

I invite you now to bring your attention all the way down to your *feet*.

You're welcome to give your feet a little wriggle if that helps you to reconnect to them.

Feel your feet contacting the floor. Begin to notice all the little sensations in your feet. Feel through your toes, the soles of your feet, the tops of your feet, around your ankles and heels. Just notice with a gentle curiosity.

Perhaps you notice feelings of pressure, tingling, softness or hardness, warmth or coolness. Whatever sensations are there, comfortable or uncomfortable, just gently notice.

And as you feel into your feet, feel the flow of your breath—just simply coming and going.

I invite you now to bring your attention to your *hands*. Feel where your hands are resting.

Notice that subtle sense of aliveness all through your hands.

And as you explore all the small sensations around and through your hands, feel the flow of your breath.

I invite you now to bring your attention to your *shoulders*. Feel into the muscles of your shoulders, starting at the base of your skull, with your muscles running down alongside your neck, across to the edges of your shoulders, and then wrapping around the front of your chest and the back of your chest, forming a diamond like shape.

What sensations can you notice? Perhaps a softness or hardness, a pressure or a tingling. Just notice the sensations, subtle or strong, with a gentle curiosity.

If you notice that your shoulders have come forward, just gently correct your posture. Gently draw your shoulder blades in and down your spine. Open your heart.

And as you feel into the muscles of your shoulders, feel the flow of your breath.

I invite you now to bring your attention to the *space in front of your eyes*. Become aware of any sensations in and around your eyes. Move your attention through your eyebrows, across your forehead. Notice whatever sensations are there.

And as you feel around the eyes and across the forehead, feel the flow of your breath.

Now open your awareness to your *whole body*—the feet, the hands, the shoulders, a little of each of these areas.

Notice whatever sensations are coming into your awareness right now—perhaps the awareness of the space in front of your eyes, perhaps the feeling of your breath. Notice the movement in the body as you inhale and as you exhale. Notice the slight pause between the inhale and the exhale—the aware mind just noticing.

(Long pause.)

If you notice your attention wandering or becoming caught up in a stream of thought, simply open your awareness. No thought is a problem; no thought is important. Worrying about your thoughts makes them heavy and important. Gently and kindly bring your attention back to the next breath. Notice sounds. Feel your feet on the floor. Feel into your hands, your shoulders. Notice the flow of your breath, the space in front of your eyes—the aware mind just noticing.

(Long pause)

Ring.

As we come towards the end of this meditation, you might like to dedicate its value and virtue and send some kind thoughts.

As we breathe in, say silently to yourself, *May I be peaceful and at ease.* As we breathe out, *May others be peaceful and at ease.* As you breathe in, allow your heart to fill with that intention, and as you breathe out, send that intention out to a group or an individual.

Breathing in, *May I be peaceful and at ease.*

Breathing out, *May others be peaceful and at ease.*

Ring.

Gently start to reactivate and re-energise your body now, perhaps with a wiggle of the fingers and toes, a deeper breath or two. You might like to have a stretch.

Bring your hands to your heart and please take a moment to thank yourself for giving yourself this time today to reconnect and recharge.

Take a final few moments to think of something you will do for yourself tomorrow—something that will help fill your cup and replenish you. It may be something as simple as going to sleep earlier or journaling three grateful things or setting some time aside to meditate. Take a moment to visualise this in your mind, hold it in your heart, and set an intention to do this for yourself tomorrow, to help fill your cup.

Thank you for joining me with this Mindfulness of Body Practice today. When you are ready, you can open your eyes.

Thank you.

Mindfulness of Emotions Practice

So, let's get our mindful bodies on. Take a few moments to find a comfortable position.

If you're sitting, sit open and upright.

Or if you're lying down, lie balanced and symmetrical. You may like to bend and support your knees to take pressure off your lower back.

Palms are open wherever they're resting.

Please close or lower your eyes.

Draw your shoulder blades in and down your spine. Open your heart space.

I invite you to take three deep belly breaths to help calm your body and mind.

Allow your body to relax and release on your exhalation. Relax and let go that little bit more with each exhalation.

Ring.

Relaxing, awake, and alert.

Remember there is nothing you need to be doing right now. There is nothing you need to experience or achieve during this Mindfulness of Emotions Practice. This is your time.

Just let your breath settle now. Let your breath breathe you.

I invite you now to bring your attention to the *space in front of your eyes.* It's like a field of darkness. Perhaps there are some muted shapes or colours there, but we're not looking for anything. We are simply resting our attention here, in this space, with relaxed eyes and a soft gaze.

I invite you now to bring your attention to any *sounds* coming from outside the room. Just listen, with a gentle curiosity.

Allow the sounds to come and go without resistance.

Now bring your attention to sounds inside the room, just listening, without judgement. Perhaps you can notice the sound of your own breath, your digestion, even your heart beating.

Allow the sounds to call you into the present moment, just listening.

I invite you to draw your attention further to your *breath*. Begin to notice any sensations associated with your breath.

Feel the slight movement of your chest and your belly.

Feel the flow of air moving past your nostrils.

Just let your breath breathe you. Follow each breath.

Allow your breath to help anchor you into the present moment.

I invite you now to bring your attention to your centre, to the feeling line of your body, from your throat all the way down to your lower pelvis.

And with the intention to check in with how you are feeling, and with a willingness to notice body sensations, gently ask yourself, *How am I feeling right now?*

Bring your attention to your *throat*. You're welcome to place a palm over your throat to help you reconnect to your throat. Feel into your throat with a gentle curiosity.

Explore any sensations, subtle or strong.

Rest your attention in the throat and allow any sensations to come into focus.

Perhaps there's a lump, a tightness, a looseness.

As you feel into your throat, feel the flow of your breath.

Now bring your attention to the *centre of your chest*, in and around your heart.

Explore any sensations there, perhaps a slight pressure, an ache, a tightness, perhaps a resistance to the breath. Or perhaps it feels soft and comfortable, an expansiveness.

Explore the body sensations free of any judgement.

As you feel into your chest, feel the flow of your breath.

Now bring your attention to your *upper belly*, your solar plexus.

Again, ask yourself, *How am I feeling right now?*

Notice any sensations in the upper belly—a softness, a tightness, a shakiness, a numbness.

Just notice any sensations with a gentle curiosity.

As you feel into your solar plexus, feel the flow of your breath.

Now bring your attention down to your *lower belly*—in, around, and behind your navel.

Notice any sensations, with a gentle curiosity.

There is no need to analyse whether the sensations come from a physical cause or an emotional cause. Just notice.

As you feel into the lower belly, feel the flow of your breath.

Now bring you attention to your *lower pelvis*, your pelvic bowl.

Notice any sensations here, just noticing without judgement.

As you feel into your lower pelvis, feel the flow of your breath.

I invite you now to open your awareness to include the *whole feeling line of your body*—your throat, chest, solar plexus, lower belly, lower pelvis.

Keep the feelings company with a gentle curiosity and compassion.

As you notice any sensations along the feeling line of your body, feel the flow of your breath.

If there is an area that feels more intense or vulnerable, gently sit with whatever sensations are there. If you begin to feel overwhelmed at any stage, please reconnect to your breath. Feel your feet on the floor. Notice sounds and/or gently open your eyes for a few moments. Let us rest here and explore the whole feeling line of the body, for a few more moments now.

(Long pause.)

If you notice your attention wandering or becoming caught up in a stream of thought, simply bring your attention back to the next breath. Feel your feet on the floor. Feel into your throat, chest, solar plexus, lower belly, and lower pelvis. Feel the flow of your breath as you are aware of the space in front of your eyes—the aware mind just noticing.

(Long pause.)

Ring.

As we come towards the end of this Mindfulness of Emotions Practice, you might like to dedicate its value and virtue and send some kind thoughts.

As we breathe in, say silently to yourself, *May I be well and happy.* As we breathe out, *May others be well and happy.* As you breathe in, allow your heart to fill with that intention and visualise yourself. As you breathe out, visualise friends, family, a group, or an individual and send that intention out to them.

Breathing in, *May I be well and happy.*

Breathing out, *May others be well and happy.*

Ring.

Gently start to reactivate and re-energise your body now, perhaps with a wiggle of the fingers and toes, a deeper breath or two. Have a little stretch. And when you're ready, you can open your eyes and go on your way.

Thank you.

FEAR Practice

The FEAR Practice was first taught to me by Pema Chodron, beloved Buddhist teacher, author, nun, and mother. This is my summary of her teaching.

Whenever you are feeling fear, embarrassment, boredom, or are on edge, the following FEAR practice can help. This can be particularly useful during the Mindfulness of Emotions Practice when more uncomfortable emotions arise. Consider using this practice whenever you experience aversion or something uncomfortable. This practice can help you learn to be gentle with yourself and to develop an unconditional friendship with yourself:

F. *Find* and *feel* the uncomfortable sensation in your body. Be present and check in, rather than checking out. (We often check out and divert our attention, particularly with constant stimulation at hand). Pause and *feel* the emotion in your body.

E. *Embrace* the feeling with kindness and gentleness. You can think of it like a small child and wrap it up in an unconditional hug.

A. *Abide* with the feeling and *allow* any associated thoughts to dissolve. Let go of any thoughts and stories. Think of the trees letting go of their leaves during autumn and winter. This allows them to conserve energy for new growth in spring.

R. *Recall* and *remember* that many other human beings all around the world have experienced, or are experiencing, this same emotion. You may have a different story, but you share the same emotion. You are not alone.

You are the sky.
Everything else—
It's just the weather.

—Pema Chodron

Mindfulness–Based Stillness Meditation (MBSM)

So, let's get our mindful bodies on. Take a few moments to adjust your posture.

If you're sitting, sit open and upright.

Or if you're lying down, lie balanced and symmetrical. You may like to bend and support your knees to take pressure off your lower back.

Palms are open wherever they are resting.

If you haven't already done so, please close or lower your eyes.

I invite you to take a wide face-stretching yawn, with an audible release on your exhalation.

Allow all the muscles of the face to soften. Allow the audible release to help you let go a little bit more.

Draw your shoulders blades in and down your spine. Open your heart space.

I invite you to take a few slow, deep belly breaths now.

As you breathe out, feel your muscles softening and relaxing. Relax and let go that little bit more with each exhalation.

Relaxing, awake and alert.

Remember there is nothing you need to be doing right now. There is nothing you need to accomplish or achieve during this Mindfulness-Based Stillness Meditation practice. This is your time.

Ring.

Allow your breath to find its own depth and rhythm now. Let your breath breathe you.

I invite you now to bring your attention to the *space in front of your eyes*. It's like a field of darkness.

Perhaps there are some muted shapes or colours there, but we're not looking for anything. Simply rest your attention there, in this space, with relaxed eyes and a soft gaze.

I invite you now to bring your attention to any *sounds* coming to you from outside the room. Just listen, with a non-judgemental curiosity.

Allow the sounds to come and go without resistance.

Now listen to sounds inside the room—just listening, without judgement. Perhaps you can notice the sound of your own breath, your digestion, even your heartbeat.

Allow the sounds to call you into the present moment, just listening.

I invite you now to draw your attention further to your *breath*. Begin to notice any sensations associated with your breath, as you breathe in and as you breathe out.

Feel the slight movement of your chest and your belly, rising with the in breath and falling with the out breath.

Feel the flow of air moving past your nostrils.

Allow the breath to help anchor you in the present moment—just your natural breath.

I invite you now to bring your attention all the way down to your *feet*. You're welcome to give your feet a little wriggle to help you reconnect to them. Begin to move your awareness through your feet.

Notice any sensations in your feet. Feel into your toes, your heels and ankles, the soles of your feet—all through the feet.

As you feel into your feet, feel the flow of your breath, simply coming and going, quite effortlessly.

I invite you now to bring your attention to your *hands*.

Notice that subtle sense of aliveness all through your hands.

As you explore all the small sensations in and around your hands, feel the flow of your breath.

I invite you now to bring your attention up to your *shoulders*.

Begin to notice any sensations in the muscles of your shoulders, perhaps a tightness, a pressure, a tingling, a warmth, a numbness. Just noticing.

Feel in and around the shoulders without judging—just simply noticing.

As you feel the muscles of your shoulders, feel the flow of your breath.

I invite you now to bring your attention to the *space in front of your eyes* again. Become aware of any sensations in and around your eyes, feel your eyelids just touching each other. Move your attention through your eyebrows and across your forehead.

Notice whatever sensations are there.

As you feel around the eyes and across the forehead, feel the flow of your breath.

I invite you now, with a willingness to get in touch with how you are feeling, to bring your awareness to your centre, *the feeling line of the body*. Most sensations associated with strong emotions are felt along the feeling line of the body—from your throat all the way down to your lower pelvis.

Gently start at your throat. Feel into your throat. Notice any sensations here and gently ask yourself, *How am I feeling right now?* As you feel in and around the throat, feel the flow of your breath.

Now feel into the centre of your chest, in and around your heart. Again, notice any sensations here. And as you feel into the heart space, feel the flow of your breath.

Now feel into the solar plexus, your upper belly—as you feel the flow of your breath.

Now feel down, around and behind your naval, into the lower belly.

Feel all the way down into the lower pelvis, the lower pelvic basin.

Just rest your attention along the whole feeling line of your body now.

Keep the feelings company with a caring and compassionate curiosity. Just simply be aware.

As you notice the sensations along the feeling line of your body, feel the flow of your breath.

I invite you to open your awareness to the whole body now.

Notice whatever sensations are coming into your awareness at this particular moment—perhaps the awareness of the space in front of your eyes, perhaps the feeling of the breath.

If any thoughts come to your awareness, just let them come when they do, and let them go when they're ready—almost like white clouds moving across a blue sky.

Watch the thoughts coming and going. Notice the background of stillness, like the blue sky, the background across which the thoughts travel—the silent presence, your true self.

Just be aware of that still and silent presence—effortlessly aware, present, watching, and listening.

Simply rest in that sense of stillness for a few moments now.

The aware mind is just noticing.

(Long pause.)

Remember, if you notice your attention wandering or becoming caught up in a stream of thought, open your awareness. Simply bring your attention back to the next breath. Feel the flow of your breath. Notice sound. Notice your feet on the floor. Notice the feeling line of your body as you rest your attention in the space in front of the eyes. And notice that still and silent presence—the aware mind just noticing.

(Long pause.)

Ring.

And now, as we come towards the end of this meditation, you may like to consciously dedicate its value and virtue and send some kind thoughts.

So, as you breathe in, say silently to yourself, *May I be well and happy.* And as you breathe out, *May others be well and happy.* Visualise yourself on your in breath and a group or an individual on your out breath.

Breathing in, *May I be well and happy.*

Breathing out, *May others be well and happy.*

Now start to reactivate and re-energise your body. Allow your breathing to become a little stronger, perhaps a deeper breath or two. You might like to wiggle your fingers and toes. Have a gentle stretch and come to a comfortable seat.

Thank you / Namaste.

MBSM Summary

Paul Bedson and Ian Gawler helpfully summarise MBSM as-[4]

Having prepared well, we relax.
Relaxing deeply, we become more mindful.
As our mindfulness develops, stillness is revealed;
naturally and without effort.
We rest in open, undistracted awareness.

Marg's Story

I have been teaching yin yoga and meditation to Marg through private sessions since 2019. In 2020, she was diagnosed with Parkinson's disease. When she shared this news with me, she appeared to be taking her diagnosis very well. When I reflected this back to her, she explained that it felt like a relief to finally have a diagnosis. She was able to understand why she had been feeling a certain way and could now do something about it.

"There is no use worrying about what I cannot change," she said.

Marg has shared that she always feels calmer, more relaxed, and in less pain following our weekly sessions together. She can now meditate without guidance. But if she starts to feel anxious or stressed, she prefers a guided meditation practice to help settle and calm her mind.

My observation is that Marg has become more confident in her practice, both physically and mentally. This is despite her Parkinson's diagnosis. She is more connected to her body and heart. She treats herself with more care and kindness. She is appreciative of her natural surroundings and of her abilities. It is an absolute pleasure and privilege to practise with her each week.

Chapter 8
Eat with the Seasons

Food has moved and evolved over time. There has been a dramatic shift in the way we process and eat food due to the agricultural revolution and then Industrial Revolution. This followed with a further desire to control the natural environment, rather than work with it, during the modern industrial age (mid nineteenth century to the present).

Mechanisation led to increased food production. Post WWI and WWII saw a shift towards large-scale use of chemical pesticides and herbicides. The majority of agricultural methods today prioritise increased production while decreasing costs. Unfortunately, this results in the quality of our food and our planet being compromised.

We currently have regimented eating patterns and are tempted to eat meals of convenience rather than sustenance. We can buy instant microwaveable meals and "fast food." We have lost connection with the true source of our foods.

Thankfully, there are changes afoot. We are learning the error of our ways. Regenerative agriculture and permaculture practices are gaining momentum. People are realising the value of acknowledging the wisdom of our ancestors and their respect for our environment. Working with the seasons and our precious planet is imperative for our survival.

Which food is best depends on the individual person, the place, and the season. There is not one specific, magical diet or ingredient that nourishes and heals everyone. There is no "one size fits all." Everybody's dietary needs differ. This is due to our different backgrounds (our heritage and genetics), life experiences, and lifestyles. These all shape our gut microbiome.

Our gut microbiome refers to all the bacteria, viruses, protozoan, fungi, and their collective genetic material present in our gastrointestinal tract. More recently, it has come to light that our gut microbiome is suffering due to heavily processed foods, pesticides, overuse of medication (particularly antibiotics), alcohol, and excess stress.

Extensive research has shown our gut microbiome is involved in maintaining our metabolism, nutrition, physiology, immune function, and mental health.[1] Eighty-five per cent of our immune system is in our gut! The communication between our gut and our brain is called the "gut-brain axis." It is a bidirectional communication system via hormones and nerves.

Several studies have found evidence of gastrointestinal inflammation and imbalance in people with depression, anxiety, bipolar disorder, and schizophrenia.[2] There is also research linking gut microbial imbalance to Parkinson's disease, other autoimmune diseases, and cardiovascular disease.[3] So, it's important to have a healthy gut microbiome! A healthy gut will support our mood regulation, mental health, physical health, and ability to connect to both ourselves and others.

If you are struggling with digestive issues, please recruit help to restore your gut microbiome. Ask trusted friends and/or family if they can recommend a good naturopath, Ayurvedic practitioner, functional medical practitioner, or other health professional.

Food can be a natural medicine to promote health and well-being. However, if the food is highly processed, full of artificial colours and flavours, and lacking in fresh energy, it can be a contributor to ill health. To quote the fantastic title of Chara Caruthers's book, you want to remember to *Eat Like You Love Yourself*.

Seasonal Eating

Seasonal eating is not new. It's the way our parents and previous generations grew up eating. Do you know what fruit and vegetables are being grown in your local area right now? Do you know what fruit and vegetables are in season?

Not only does eating seasonally help you reconnect to the seasons and to your local environment, it also allows you to eat fresh food. The fresher the food, the more nutritional value and taste it has. The fruit, vegetables, and other foods that are available during each season are the very foods we need. They contain exactly what we need to promote and maintain our health during that season.

Research studies show that the phytonutrients present in raw fruit and vegetables are altered during cold storage. A fresh, locally grown piece of broccoli has a much higher vitamin C level than an imported piece of broccoli. This is due to the former having spent less or no time in cold storage and endured less travel time. So, the ideal way to eat our fruit and vegetables is as fresh as possible. We want to be able to access the potent antioxidants they contain when they're fresh in order to maintain and/or improve our health and immunity.

By eating seasonally, you also provide yourself with a diverse range of foods. You eat variety with each season, delivering the right nutrients at the right time in the right place. Seasonal food is easily available and optionally nutritious. A general rule of thumb is, whatever is fresh, abundant, and affordable at the market is what is in season.

PIP Magazine, an Australian permaculture magazine designed to help you nourish yourself, your community, and the planet puts it this way: "When we choose to eat what is in season and to eat locally grown foods, we reduce or remove the harmful and wasteful aspects of processing, packaging, transport, storage and additives, and we begin to take control of what we eat."

So, to sum it up, seasonal food is more cost-effective, tastes better, involves less waste, and provides us with the nutrients we need during each season.

Yin and Yang of Food

TCM believes different foods affect the way our organs interact with our chi flow, our mind, and our emotions. Food is natural medicine. It can promote our health and well-being. Fresh food is rich in chi, whereas heavily processed food with a long shelf life, is low in chi.

As the weather changes with the seasons, we dress appropriately to accommodate. We wear fewer clothes in summer to keep cool and more clothes in winter to keep warm. We can do the same with our choice of food and cooking method each season. We can eat foods that keep us internally cool in summer and warm in winter. By responding to our environment, we can avoid its extremes and maintain our own internal balance.

Yin foods are cooling foods, and yang foods are warming. Plants that grow quickly are considered more cooling, such as lettuce, radish, cucumber, and zucchini. Plants that take longer to grow are considered more warming such as carrot, cabbage, parsnip, and ginseng.

So, in the warmer yang seasons of spring and summer, we want to eat more yin foods to maintain balance. All the cooling yin vegetables are perfect for making delicious salads. Eating raw food is more cooling than eating cooked food. The cooling yin foods are seasonally available during the warmer months.

In the cooler yin seasons of autumn and winter, we want to eat more yang foods to create warmth. Slow-cooked root vegetables, soups, and stews are warming and nourishing. The yang foods are seasonally available during the cooler months. How wonderful that the fruits and vegetables that are available during each season are exactly the foods we need to promote and maintain our health.

Cooking methods impart warming properties to food. There is a sliding scale of warmth imparted; a quick stir-fry will impart less warmth than a slow-cooked stew. We will go into further detail about cooking methods and types of food in the individual seasonal practice chapters found in Part II of this book.

Growing Food

A powerful way to connect to your local seasons is to start growing your own food. I grew up eating seasonally whenever I stayed with my dad and stepmum; of course, it didn't have a label back then. We grew a vegetable garden and many tropical fruit trees. We kept chickens, pigs, a horse, and goats. I used to milk the goat.

I have happy memories of digging up the golden treasure of fresh sweet potatoes and of carefully cracking open macadamia nuts and eating them straight out of their hard shell. There was simple pleasure involved in picking and eating fresh tropical fruit straight from the trees.

By growing some of your own food or flowers you become even more attuned to the seasons. Getting your hands into the soil, watching the plants grow, carefully picking the garden gifts, and eating them—these all contribute to connection. Even better, when you have a surplus, you can share or swap it with friends and neighbours and create further connection.

I experience such a sense of wonder, connection, and calm when I spend time in a garden. I do even more so when I'm picking, collecting, and harvesting fruit, vegetables, and flowers. There is a sense of wonder and awe at what mother earth can produce and gift us with.

This morning, I spent fifteen minutes picking beans from the beanstalks wound along our pool fence. I took time to gently lift the leaves and discover what wonders lay underneath. I found baby beans, mummy-size beans, and daddy-size beans. I carefully picked suitably sized beans, without pulling too much on the plant. I noticed the flowers and the busy insects interspersed between the bean plants. There were small delicate bean flowers, green leaves, golden marigolds, and deep red nasturtiums, all offering a palate of colour. There was one small snail, many busy-looking ants, and a cabbage moth fluttering about. I experienced an informal mindful moment in the garden.

I appreciate that not everyone has the space, time, and strength for growing a vegetable garden, flowers, or fruit trees. Other alternatives and suggestions to help you attune to the seasons through food are:

- Brighten up the inside of your home by treating yourself to a bunch of seasonal flowers. Pick them yourself or find a local florist to support.
- Grow your own herbs. This can be done in a pot; you don't need a backyard.
- Buy from your local farmers' market or direct from the farm door. Both options connect you directly to the farmers whilst you purchase seasonally.
- Have a weekly seasonal fruit and vegetable box delivered.
- Discuss what is in season with your local greengrocer. Or you can use Google to find out what fruit, vegetables, and meats are currently in season where you live.
- Eat home-cooked meals made with seasonal produce.

As I am currently living in Melbourne/Naarm, the seasonal food section in the seasonal practice chapters will be Victoria-centric. I encourage you to find out what local fruit and vegetables are in season near you.

Nina's Story

My adventurous friend Nina and I have known each other for over twenty years. We lived together in London many moons ago and travelled through Europe together. She started attending my classes and workshops in 2020.

Nina shared with me that she had a patch in her life where everything felt like it came undone. There was a slow death occurring in her family. She was working hard, caring for her two daughters, and supporting her husband in starting up his own business.

She started having strange and unsettling neurological signs and symptoms—head tension that felt like someone was squeezing her skull, sensitive skin, dizziness to the point of being unable to walk easily, exhaustion, regularly waking at 3:00 a.m. with heart palpitations, and teeth grinding.

Appointments with her GP plus numerous investigative tests resulted in a diagnosis of anxiety. Once Nina was given the diagnosis, she took it on board and decided to get well and to look after herself.

Nina has learned it is most empowering to have a toolkit. Nina's toolkit includes:

- Meditation
- Yoga
- Supportive health professionals
- Gardening

My garden also helps me think spiritually. It offers a direct connection to nature. Being outside, having space and sky and sun. All the things that nourish you. Every morning I'm outside with my cup of tea in the garden. I've never been a particularly patient person. In the past I have always wanted things in a hurry. I've been fast-moving and on the go. There is absolutely no room for that in the garden; you just have to be patient. The life lessons I have learned through my garden have been amazing. I might transplant tender seedlings into the garden and then come out to find them all eaten overnight by slugs. I have learned to watch, learn, recover, and start again.

—Nina

Permaculture Principles

The production process and the type of food we eat impacts not only our health but also the health of our planet. In the table below I share with you the positive principles of a permaculture diet, which suitably follows the acronym HEALS.

Healthy

Use food in which both the production process and the effect of eating the food are beneficial to health. Food produced with care is best, so choose animals and plants that are well looked after—for example, organic produce.

Ethical

The permaculture ethics are *people care, earth care, and fair share*. Food you have produced yourself or food that comes from local sources and/or from ethical businesses are best–for example, fair trade options.

Alive

Choose food that's fresh and "alive"—fruit and vegetables that look, feel, and smell fresh. Avoid foods that are limp, overly processed, and lacking in colour and flavour.

Local

Choose food that has travelled less. It is fresher, has used less fossil fuel, and supports your local community. Increased interest in local food is one of the positive changes of recent times.

Seasonal

Food that is in season is fresh and full of nutrients. Cold-stored food has often been picked unripe, has limited flavour and nutrients, and has travelled far. If you desire certain flavours out of season, consider more conscientious ways to consume them. In other words, look for locally sourced, salt-preserved lemons, jam, dehydrated mushrooms and fruit, and garlic oil.

Reducing waste is also an important aspect of the permaculture principles. We can do this by using the whole animal, preserving and fermenting excess food in season, and using minimal packaging. Less waste results in less damage to the planet, and we get more from the food we do have.

General Dietary Suggestions for Vitality and Well-being

For vitality and well-being:
1. Eat seasonally.
2. Avoid eating late at night.
3. Avoid sudden, extreme diet changes. Gradual change is best.
4. Relax while eating. Breathe deeply and chew thoroughly. Deep breaths help trigger our PNS into rest, *digest*, heal, and grow mode.
5. Give thanks before and/or after your meal.
6. Avoid overeating.
7. Prioritise whole natural foods.
8. Eat more vegetables than fruit. Eat plenty of green, leafy vegetables and cruciferous vegetables. Examples of cruciferous vegetables are broccoli, Brussels sprouts, bok choy, broccolini, mustard greens, watercress, broccoli sprouts, and cauliflower. Cruciferous vegetables are particularly helpful for women, as they help reduce excess oestrogen, along with decreasing inflammation and regulating blood sugar.
9. Eat berries, nuts, and seeds.

10. If you eat meat and dairy, choose to buy from ethical suppliers. This means the suppliers take into consideration the welfare of the animals involved and use sustainable farming practices. For example, choose local grass-fed beef. Avoid meat from unhappy animals full of hormones and antibiotics. This also includes fish. Look for locally sourced and sustainably caught fish. Eat meat and dairy in moderation.

11. Limit/avoid weakening foods such as refined sugar and its products, intoxicants such as coffee and alcohol, too much salt, and overly processed food.

12. Consume good quality oil and fats. Which oil is best has been discussed and debated for years. The type of oil you consume impacts the level of inflammation in your body. Corn, peanut, soya bean, vegetable, canola, and seed oils all contain unstable fats that can contribute to inflammation. Avoid trans fats; they're found in fried and greasy foods and have been shown to be associated with obesity, heart disease, high cholesterol, and oestrogen imbalance. A good quality olive oil, coconut oil, grass-fed butter and ghee, and MCT oil are healthy oils and fats. (MCT stands for medium chain triglyceride, a group of fatty molecules that are relatively small and, therefore, easy for the body to absorb and process for energy.) Other good fats are avocados, fish oil, cacao butter, and dark chocolate.

13. Consume bone broth (if you are not vegan, vegetarian and/or don't have histamine intolerance). Bone broth is packed full of anti-inflammatory proteins, amino acids, and minerals. It contains gelatin, glycine, glucosamine, chondroitin, arginine, and glutamine. These all contribute to the health of our hair, skin, bones, and joints. They also help to heal the gut and aid digestion.

14. Include foods rich in minerals in your diet. Some of the richest and most complete sources are seaweeds, such as kelp, kombu, and wakame.

15. Eating sprouted grains, legumes, and seeds is ideal, particularly in the warmer months. Sprouting results in the fats, proteins, and starches being broken down into more easily digested forms.

Please remember to avoid certain foods if you are allergic or intolerant to them, even if they are listed as a food to prioritise.

Fasting

"Fasting"
There's hidden sweetness in the stomach's emptiness.
We are lutes, no more, no less. If the soundbox
is stuffed full of anything, no music.
If the brain and the belly are burning clean
with fasting, every moment a new song comes out of the fire.
The fog clears, and new energy makes you
run up the steps in front of you.
Be emptier and cry like reed instruments cry.
Emptier, write secrets with the reed pen.
When you're full of food and drink, an ugly metal
statue sits where your spirit should. When you fast,
good habits gather like friends who want to help.
Fasting is Solomon's ring. Don't give it
to some illusion and lose your power,
but even if you have, if you've lost all will and control,
they come back when you fast, like soldiers appearing
out of the ground, pennants flying above them.
A table descends to your tents,
Jesus' table.
Expect to see it, when you fast, this table
spread with other food, better than the broth of cabbages.

—Rumi[4]

Fasting is going without or abstaining from something. It doesn't always relate to food. For example, you could go without alcohol and drugs, and this is called sobriety. Or you could go without gadgets and screens, and this is called a screen detox. We are going to focus on fasting in relation to food in this book.

The practice of deliberate fasting dates back thousands of years. Indigenous Aboriginal Elders would take the young people out to fast in order to help them find their direction in life. It is also a central element of Ayurveda, the system of health developed in India three thousand years ago. Almost every world religion advocates a period of fasting to attain spiritual enlightenment.

Fasting helps us to develop discipline and self-control. It helps detox the body, reduce inflammation, and clear the mind. It also helps us develop compassion. When we fast, we experience some of the hunger others are unwillingly enforced to endure. Letting go of our focus on food can free up time for other things and improve our relationship with food.

Over the past few years, I have experimented with a few fasting variations. I have found intermittent fasting to be particularly helpful and healing for me, so I share further details here.

The 16:8 fast is when you consume your food within a shortened time period (typically around eight hours) and fast for the rest of the time (sixteen hours). The easiest way to do this is to skip breakfast, break your fast at around noon, and then stop eating for the day at around 8:00 p.m.

Fast This Way: Burn Fat, Heal Inflammation and Eat Like the High-Performing Human You Were Meant to Be by David Asprey is a great resource and guide if you are just starting out with fasting. Dave has spent years researching and trying many various methods of fasting himself. Choose to fast in a way that makes sense to you and resonates with your body, mind, and heart.

Dave suggests one crucial biohack to make your intermittent fast of 16:8 (or longer) easier and more effective: "Drink a cup of Bulletproof Coffee in the morning."[5] I don't drink coffee, as it inflames my nervous system. I like to drink a cup of good quality, ethical drinking cacao with MCT oil added instead.

Archbishop Desmond Tutu fasted on a weekly basis for many, many years. As he grew older, his doctors advised him to drink during his fast, so he began having "hot chocolate fasts." I love this. I am a big fan of intermittent fasting with ceremonial-grade drinking cacao. Along with the health benefits of both the quality cacao and the fasting, I also gain a clear energy boost and more access to creativity. Fasting fact—I have used intermittent fasting with cacao to write most of this book.

Among fasting's many benefits, it:
- Makes your body burn fat
- Helps your gut heal itself
- Evokes the body's self-cleaning system (autophagy) and detoxification process
- Reduces your risk of almost every chronic disease
- Causes your body to produce more stem cells
- Reduces your risk of type 2 diabetes by improving insulin sensitivity
- Slows aging from oxidative stress
- Reduces inflammation
- Boosts your emotional state
- Improves your relationship with food
- Improves mental clarity
- Enhances your ability to enter a spiritual and meditative state
- Enhances creativity

It's important to note that fasting impacts the female body differently than it does the male body. Men and women have different hormone levels, and this results in them requiring different dietary patterns. Historically, most research on fasting has been done on men; hence, most fasting guidelines have been developed for men. Please remember that, as women, we are designed for childbearing, so we are more sensitive to shortfalls in energy.

If women fast too much, it can send a stress signal to the body—"Emergency! There is a famine. Don't reproduce." As a result, a rapid decline in sex hormones can occur. This can lead to irregular periods, temporary infertility, hair loss, sleeplessness/insomnia, anxiety, and poor bone health. It's important to learn to listen to your body and not take fasting too far.

As women, we can still gain all the benefits of fasting without compromising our health; we just need to make some modifications.

Some important intermittent fasting guidelines for females include:

- Don't intermittent fast every day.
- Women are more susceptible to becoming addicted to intermittent fasting; signs of taking fasting too far include hair loss, decreased sleep quality, adrenal exhaustion, menstrual cycle changes, anxiety, poor bone health and even temporary infertility.
- Don't exercise too heavily or do high-intensity interval training whilst intermittent fasting.
- Never fast when pregnant.
- Don't fast if you are underweight, have a history of an eating disorder, or are anaemic.
- Don't fast if you are recovering from an illness or are unwell.
- Don't intermittent fast during your period or the few days prior; this is when your metabolism is high and you need more energy.
- If you are perimenopausal try shorter intermittent fasts and don't do them back to back until you are sure they are working/good for you.
- There is a tremendous range in the way women's bodies respond at and after menopause, so your response to fasting will also change.
- Please check in with your GP before fasting, particularly if you have an underlying health condition.
- Listen to your body. Signs of adrenal exhaustion may include craving salty and fatty foods. Try adding some good quality salt (Himalayan, Murray River salt) and healthy fats into your diet and take a break from fasting for a while. A water element nourishing practice (found in Chapter 11)) will also help.
- The yang seasons of the year, spring, summer, and late summer, are naturally more conducive to fasting. Be cautious with fasting during the yin seasons of autumn and winter, as this is a time when our body needs to reserve energy.

Healing Cacao

All foods don't suit everyone, as discussed earlier, and cacao is no exception. I have friends and past patients who suffer terribly from migraines following cacao ingestion. But I have personally found good quality cacao so helpful and healing that I am including some information here. You can choose whether to investigate further.

My positive experiences with cacao have involved both the cacao products and the women behind their production, Nicole Trutanich based in the United States, and Fipe Preuss based in Australia.

I was first introduced to the magic of chocolate by the chocolate princess (as she is affectionately known in our family), Nicole Trutanich, in 2011. Prior to this, I wasn't that much of a chocolate fan, and I actually didn't like chocolate bars at all as a kid.

I met Nicole in Oaxaca whilst my family and I were travelling around Mexico, and she was travelling for work. She was sourcing cacao farmers who use traditional and sustainable harvesting, fermenting, and drying techniques. Nicole was in the early stages of running her chocolate business, Bar Au' Chocolat. Nicole passionately educated me and my family on the merits of chocolate. We shared laughs, stories, and Día de los Muertos celebrations together in Mexico. Most importantly, we explored good quality Mexican chocolate together, and our friendship was sealed.

True dark chocolate (not the mass-produced, artificial flavoured, and coloured confectionary kind) has wonderful healing and ceremonial properties. Lots of research now supports this. I have highlighted some research findings below.

Among cacao's positive healing properties, it:

- Is rich in polyphenols, which improve the gut microbiome and brain health and protect against heart disease, type 2 diabetes, and even certain cancers

- Is a significant source of magnesium
- Improves nitric oxide levels
- Has been shown to reduce inflammation (by reducing C-reactive protein)
- Enhances cardiovascular health
- Protects the brain, reducing age and disease-related cognitive decline
- Reduces asthmatic episodes linked to inflammation

Good quality cacao, with its bitter taste, is renowned as a medicine of the heart in many cultures around the world. In TCM, it is believed to impact the Heart, Liver, and Kidney meridians. Therefore, cacao influences emotional balance, heart-led action, harmonious flow of chi, digestive function, body repair and maintenance, fluid balance and ageing. I always have a pot of cacao husk tea ready in the studio for participants of my classes. And when leading retreats or workshops I often share ceremonial grade drinking cacao.

Fipe's Story

My warm-hearted friend Fipe Preuss comes from a family of Samoan cacao growers. Her grandfather was the high chief of the district. He created his own strand of cacao by grafting two main species of cacao together. His aim was to create a stronger more disease-resistant strand, which he called Lafi7. (Lafi was the name of the area he was grafting and planting on; seven is the number of attempts it took him to get the best bean quality.) He encouraged and activated many people to cultivate their own domestic cacao plots in Samoa.

Cacao is richly embedded in the Samoan culture. It is regularly brewed up as a potent hot drink to be shared with friends and family. Cacao encourages an opening of the heart and deep *talanoa*. Talanoa is the Samoan word for conversation. Cacao offers deep, truthful conversation with self and others.

"*Koko* in Samoan means cacao, but *koko*, also known as *toto*, means blood," Fipe explains.

Following the loss of a dear friend in 2012, Fipe was left feeling heartbroken. Fipe realised that, if she wanted to start seeing light again, she needed to make some changes. She needed to create spaces of light for herself and to remember that there was beauty in the world. Cacao was a huge part of this.

Fipe created Living Koko with her partner Glen Reiss in 2015. Living Koko creates small-batch, guilt-free cacao indulgence. The cacao beans are sourced through an organisation called Savaii Koko. Savaii works directly with a network of women domestic plot farmers who use sustainable farming methods. They provide fair and ethical trade. Living Koko provides Fipe and Glen with a way of supporting communities back home in Samoa and also supporting communities here in Melbourne. Their cacao products are magical and full of wonder.

Whilst recently nurturing herself with her own cacao ceremony, Fipe recently gained this insight, and she has graciously agreed for me to share it here. I hope you find it helpful:

*I have never been good at loving myself. I used to think I was good at loving people but realised
what I thought was love was my need to please people for my own self-worth.
I know this as I have kept quiet through betrayal.
I know this as I smile still at those that have hurt me.
I know this as I have ignored the signs and people's toxic patterns.
But I'm seeing it all now. I am seeing what is truly for me and my own patterns. I see, I sit in it, and release with love.
My heart is open, I am aware … and I am grateful for the lessons.*

—Fipe

Part II

Seasonal Practices

Chapter 9

Autumn

Autumn is traditionally a time of harvest. It's a time to collect and gather, both internally and externally. It's a time to plan and prepare for the approaching stillness of winter.

Have you noticed your natural surroundings during autumn? The days begin to grow shorter, and the natural light is softer. There's a sharp coolness each evening and morning. Many leaves turn into an awe-inspiring palette of red, gold, and amber before starting to fall. The trees show us how easy and beautiful it is to let things go.

Leaves and fruit fall, seeds dry, and tree sap moves down into the roots. Everything in nature contracts and moves its essence inward and downward. Internally, our own bodies also bring energy inwards and downwards during autumn.

Externally, we stock up on warm clothing, fuel, and food. It's a time for harvesting crops. During autumn, yin grows, and yang subsides.

As the temperature drops and it turns cooler, we're naturally drawn towards snuggling up and staying indoors. We tend to want to go out less and socialise less. This can help to quieten our mind. It is easier to turn towards more contemplative and slower practices during this time. We naturally turn inwards and towards the practice of *svadhyaya* (self-inquiry and self-study).

Autumn corresponds to the metal element in TCM (five element theory). The metal element involves our Lung and Large Intestine meridians. These meridians are believed to be more vulnerable during autumn.

In TCM, the Lung and Large Intestine meridians have a big role in immunity, respiration (mainly expiration), nourishment, vocal expression, and the balance of moisture in the body.

The metal element is associated with the emotions of grief, sadness, and yearning. When we experience excessive grief, this can drain or deplete our metal element. And vice versa, if our metal element is blocked or imbalanced, then we are more prone to persistent grief or to not being able to feel grief at all. We can feel numb and without emotion; we can feel stuck and blocked. This can develop into depression and melancholy. When our metal element is balanced and in harmony, then we can let go of what no longer serves us.

Those with metal element balance:
- Are courageous and reverent
- Are effective in how they go about their tasks and maintain purpose
- Are able to let go of what is no longer helpful or is unnecessary
- Express awe and wonder easily

Those with metal element imbalance may experience:
- Respiratory disorders—coughs, bronchitis, chest pain
- An inability to take in on many levels, with symptoms such as allergies, asthma, skin rashes, and hives
- Neck and shoulder pain/problems
- Constipation, dry stools
- Dry and/or itchy skin, dry nose, dry lips, dry mouth
- Frequent thirst
- A weak voice
- Feeling excessive or persistent grief
- Feeling stuck or dogmatically positioned
- An inability to experience grief, feeling "stopped up" or blocked
- Resistance to cold and dry environments

The poems, practices, and food suggestions in this chapter are all shared here to help support and nourish your metal element. This is important in the one to two weeks leading up to and during autumn. The suggested asana sequence, pranayama and meditation practices are also helpful throughout the year if you are experiencing any of the aforementioned signs and symptoms of imbalance.

During the metal nourishing asana sequence, we focus on sensation in the arms and shoulders. It's helpful to focus on physically and emotionally "letting go" during this metal element nourishing practice, just like the trees. Can you allow your body to let go? Can you allow your muscles to gently relax and release a little more with each exhalation? Can you allow your mind to let go of any thoughts clamouring for your attention? Can you let go of your to-do list? Can you let go of any roles or habitual patterns that no longer serve you?

Beneficial Autumn Food and Preparation

During autumn, aim to use cooking methods that involve more focused preparation to supply more energy. In general, we want to cook at a lower heat and for longer periods of time. This results in our food being more easily digested. As the weather turns colder, start to eat more soups, stews, porridge, and slow-cooked meals. It's time to dust off your slow cooker and put it to work all through autumn and into the coming winter.

Start to replace raw and cold foods, eaten during the warmer seasons, with cooked and warm foods. Stay hydrated with warm water and herbal teas, rather than cold drinks.

As energy moves downwards during autumn, it is helpful to eat foods with downward energy such as seasonal root vegetables. These include potatoes, carrots, parsnips, sweet potatoes, swedes, and turnips. Concentrated foods and root vegetables help to thicken the blood during the cooler weather.

The metal element corresponds to the nose and our sense of smell. We can stimulate our appetite with the warm fragrance of baked and sautéed food during autumn. Add warming spices like ginger, cardamom, cinnamon, pepper, and chilli to your meals.

In TCM, foods that are naturally white in colour are also said to nourish our metal element. So autumn is the time to enjoy radish, white cabbage, horseradish, cauliflower, and onion.

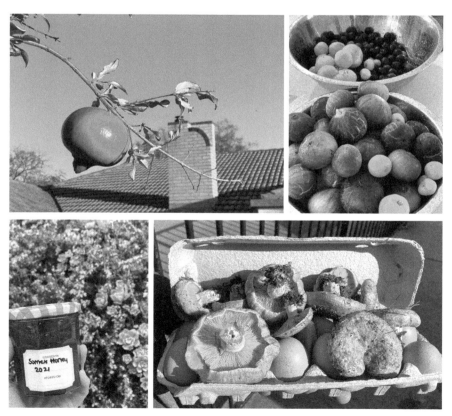

Metal Element Nourishment

Meridian Tapping and Acupressure

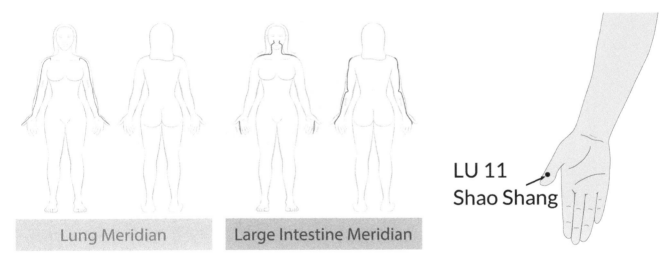

Lung Meridian

Large Intestine Meridian

LU 11
Shao Shang

Lung Meridian

The external Lung meridians start in the hollow regions in front of the shoulders. They then run down the inside of the outer arms, through the wrists, and down to the inside tip of the thumbs. There is a small internal branch each side, which connects to the tip of the index fingers, where the Large Intestine meridians start.

LU 11 Shao Shang / Lesser Shang

These acupressure points are found at the outer end of the thumbnails. When stimulated, they can help sore throats, nosebleeds, cough, and asthma. We can gently direct pressure through the thumb tips, and hence these acupressure points, when practising Cat/Cow in the metal element nourishing sequence below.

Large Intestine Meridian

The external Large Intestine meridians start at the tips of the index fingers. They then run up along the outside of the arms to the shoulders and up along the sides of the neck. From here they travel over the jaw, curve around the upper lips, and cross over to the opposite side to finish at the edges of the nose. They are the only meridians to cross over the midline of the body.

Wonder Full Poem and Quote

"A Necessary Autumn Inside Each"

You and I have spoken all these words,
but as for the way we have to go,
words are no preparation.
There is no getting ready, other than grace ...
Inside each of us, there's continual autumn.
Our leaves fall and are blown out over the water.
A crow sits in the blackened limbs
and talks about what's gone ...
There's a necessary dying,
and then Jesus is breathing again.
Very little grows on jagged rock.
Be ground. Be crumbled, so wildflowers
will come up where you are.
You've been stony for too many years.
Try something different.
Surrender.

—Rumi[1]

The three months of Fall are called the period of tranquillity of one's conduct ... Soul and spirit should be gathered together in order to make the breath of Fall tranquil ... all of this is the protection of one's harvest. In the autumn all things in creation approach their harvest, perfection and completion.

—Lao Tzu, *Tao Te Ching*[2]

Intention for Practice

As you begin, please take a moment to pause and set your intention for practice today.
For example:

I intend to cultivate mindful attention towards my body with its breath, my heart, and my mind during today's practice.

I will nourish my metal element through certain movement, pranayama, words, and meditation.

I will pay particular attention to the ancient energy lines of the Lung and Large Intestine meridians. Where our attention goes, our energy flows. I will practise asanas that stretch, squash, and squeeze along the Lung and Large Intestine meridians.

As I practise today, it is inclusive of all feelings, sensations, and circumstances as they arise. I will guide my attention with a gentle curiosity, an open heart, and kindness.

Beneficial Metal Element Meditation Practices

▷ Mindfulness of Body Practice, highlighting Lung and Large Intestine meridians (chapter 7)
▷ Mindfulness of Breath Practice (chapter 7)
▷ Harvest and nourish ourselves with a gratitude practice (chapter 4)
▷ Mindfulness of Emotions Practice (chapter 7)
▷ MBSM (chapter 7)

Practice Dedication

Finish with dedicating the value and virtue of your practice and sending kind thoughts.
For example:

> As I come towards the end of this practice, I would like to dedicate its value and virtue and send some kind thoughts.

> As I breathe in, *May I be filled with grace and gratitude.* As I breathe out *May [he, she, they] be filled with grace and gratitude.*

As you breathe in, allow your heart to fill with this intention and visualise yourself. As you breathe out, visualise an individual or a group of people and send that intention out to them. Practise this for three breaths.

Next, come to a comfortable seated position, bring your hands into a prayer position in front of your heart, and gently bow your head into anjali mudra. Take a moment to thank yourself for giving yourself the time and space to practise this morning, to attune to autumn, and to fill your cup.

Bring your thumbs to your third eye centre as a gesture of honour, respect, and gratitude to yourself, to others, and to the practice experienced today. And close with, "thank you/namaste."

Beneficial Metal Element Sequence

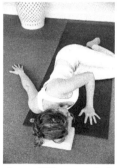

Body tapping down LU & up LI meridians 3 times each, avoid if pregnant

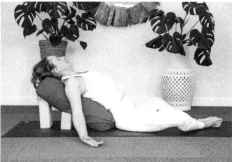

Supported Fish / Thoracic Bridge plus set intention for practice whilst belly breathing (3-5 minutes)

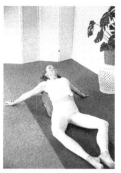

Supported Lounging Monkey (1-2 minutes)

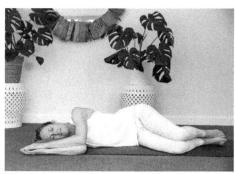

Side-lying Rebound plus long exhale breath (1 minute)

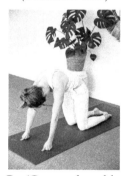

Open Wings on left and then right side (2 minutes each)

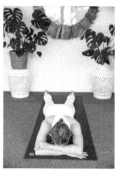

Prone Rebound (30-60 seconds)

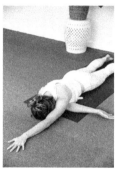

Embracing Wings on left and then right side (2 minutes each)

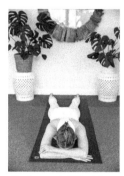

Prone Rebound (30-60 seconds)

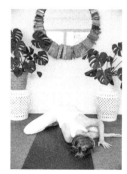

Cat/Cow on knuckles with thumbs out for LU11 stimulation (1 minute)

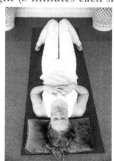

Wide-legged Child's Pose with twist to left and then right (3 minutes each side)

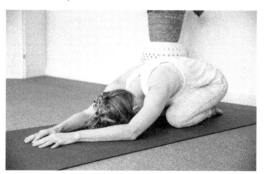

Child's Pose plus ujjayi breath (1 minute)

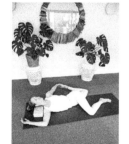

Cat Pulling Tail on right then left (3 minutes each side) with Rebound in between sides

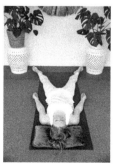

Side-lying/CPR/Savasana rebound (1 minute)

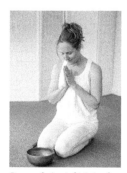

Savasana/CRP/comfortable seated position for chosen meditation

Seated Anjali Mudra plus dedication

Chapter 10
Winter

Winter is a time of hibernation, when we feel naturally drawn to snuggling up and staying indoors. Energy moves inwards during winter. It's a time of yin. It's a time to increase our self-care. It's a time to rest, to meditate deeply, and to refine our spiritual practice. The ability to listen deeply is heightened during winter's cold, silent months.

Winter corresponds to the water element in TCM (five elements theory). The water element involves our Kidney and Urinary Bladder meridians. These meridians are considered more vulnerable during this season.

The Kidneys are considered the gate of life and store *jing*, our very essence, our vital energy. The Kidney and Urinary Bladder meridians need to remain balanced for all the other organs to function well.

Our jing is depleted by stress, fear, insecurity, and overwork. It is also depleted by toxins, too much dietary protein, and excessive sweet food. There seems to be an excess of most or all of these in our modern lifestyle at present. As Paul Pitchford notes in *Healing with Whole Foods*, "While other seasons and organs demand a balance, it is almost impossible to be too good to the Kidneys."[1]

So, regardless of the season, it's important to include Kidney nourishing poses in each mindful movement practice. Good nutrition is important for building and maintaining our jing. Towards the end of this chapter, you will find a section called "Beneficial Food and Preparation" specifically for nourishing our water element in winter.

The primary function of the water element meridians is to govern our water metabolism, longevity, reproduction, physical development, emotional maturity, and bone strength. They also provide energy and warmth. Our longevity is directly related to our Kidney meridian health. So, as we age it becomes increasingly more important to spend time and attention nourishing our water element.

The water element is associated with the emotions of fear, dread, insecurity, and paralysed will. When we experience excessive fear, this can drain or deplete our water element. And vice versa, if our water element is weak or imbalanced, then we will be more prone to feeling fear and dread. This in turn can block loving and joyful experiences.

Those with balanced water element:
- Are dependable and clear thinking
- Are active yet calm
- Are courageous and gentle
- Have strong bones, hair, and teeth
- Mature gracefully

Those with water element imbalance may experience:
- Bone problems, especially knees, lower back, and teeth
- Ear problems, such as hearing loss, ear infections/diseases, and tinnitus
- Head and/or hair problems, including hair loss, split ends, and premature greying
- Urinary problems. like incontinence, bed-wetting, and urinary retention
- Sexual and reproductive imbalance, low sex drive
- Bad hot flushes in perimenopause and menopause
- Premature ageing
- Feelings of excessive fear, paralysed will, timidity, dread, and insecurity
- Poor growth and development of the mind and body
- Moving from one problem to the next without recognising the cause of the problem(s)
- Difficulty thinking clearly, poor memory, and/or early dementia

The poems, practices, and food suggestions included in this chapter are to help support and nourish your water element. This is important in the one to two weeks leading up to and during winter. The suggested asana sequence, pranayama and meditation practices are also helpful throughout the year if you are experiencing any of the aforementioned signs and symptoms of imbalance.

During the water element nourishing asana sequence, we focus on backbends and forward bends. All backbends and forward bends influence the Kidney and Urinary Bladder meridians.

Beneficial Foods and Preparation

In winter, we need to eat foods to create warmth. Warming soups and stews are perfect for this. Get your slow cooker working for you regularly. Fill it with seasonal vegetables and a good quality source of protein. During winter, we want to cook foods longer, at lower temperatures, and with less water. Storing physical energy in the form of a little added body weight during winter also helps to create warmth.

Bone broth is particularly warming and nourishing during the yin seasons of autumn and winter (provided you are not vegan or vegetarian or have histamine intolerance.) If you are experiencing an upset digestion, bone broth can be particularly helpful and healing.

Nuts are a winter food. They protect themselves with hard shells and leathery outer husks. They are designed to be carried and stored inside, waiting to be eaten during colder times. They are full of good healthy fat and protein, and delicious heavy calories to keep you warm.

Both bitter and salty foods promote a sinking, centring quality appropriate during winter. They encourage heat to move deeper and lower. Bitter flavours, such as good quality cacao, nourish and protect the heart-mind connection. Always use salt with care. Salty foods include miso, tamari, soy sauce, seaweeds, good quality salt, and foods with added salt.

Black or dark-coloured food (and clothing) nourishes the water element and conserve jing. Foods that tone and direct energy to the Kidneys in general are black beans cooked with a little seaweed and a pinch of salt, millet, wheat, black sesame seeds, chestnuts, walnuts, nettles, bee pollen, and royal jelly.

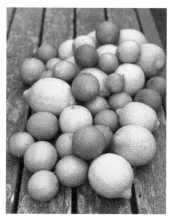 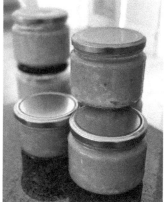 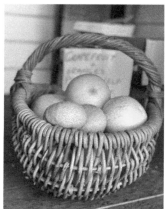 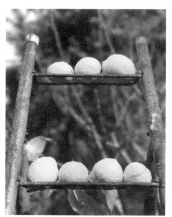

Victorian Winter Produce

Fruit—apples, avocado, grapefruit, lemon, lime, mandarin, orange, pear

Herbs & Edible Flowers—bay leaf, calendula, lemon balm, parsley, thyme, rosemary

Vegetables—beetroot, bok choy, broccoli, broad bean, Brussels sprout, cabbage, carrot, celery, cauliflower, Jerusalem artichoke, leek, parsnip, potato, fennel, spinach, turnip

Water Element Nourishment

Meridian Tapping and Acupressure

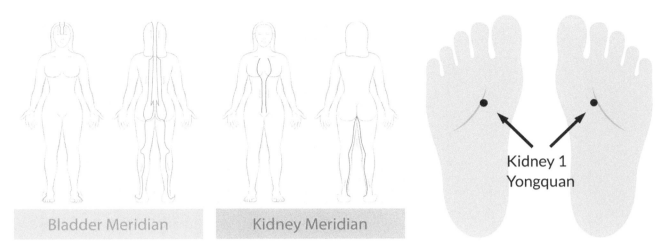

Bladder Meridian   Kidney Meridian   Kidney 1 Yongquan

Urinary Bladder Meridian

The external Urinary Bladder meridians are the longest in the body. They are like a superhighway that runs along the posterior (back) fascial line of the body. They start at the inner corner of both eyes, run up over the forehead and over the back of the head, extend parallel alongside the spine down to the buttocks and along the back of the legs to the outer ankles, and finish in the small toes.

Kidney Meridian

The external Kidney meridians start at the small toes, near the end of the Urinary Bladder meridians. They travel across the bottom of the centre of the feet, up the inner lower leg, inner knee, and inner thighs and to the base of the spine. They flow from either side of the pubic bone and up the abdomen and chest to finish at the inner side of the clavicles/collarbones.

KD 1 Yongquan / Gushing Spring

These acupuncture points are located on the soles of the feet between the second and third toes at the top third of the feet. When stimulated, they are grounding and calming. They can help relieve headaches, hypertension, low back pain, anxiety, insomnia, nausea, hot flushes, and night sweats. We can massage these points during our water element nourishing practice.

Wonder Full Poem and Quote

In the midst of chaos, I found there was, within me, an invincible calm. In the midst of winter, I found there was, within me, an invincible summer. And that makes me happy. For it says that no matter how hard the world pushes against me, within me, there's something stronger—something better, pushing right back."
—Albert Camus, *The Stranger*[2]

Intention for Water Element Nourishing Practice

As you begin, please take a moment to pause and set your intention for practice today.
For example:

> I intend to cultivate mindful attention towards my body with its breath, my heart, and my mind during today's practice.

> I will nourish my water element through certain mindful movement, pranayama, words, and meditation.

> I will pay particular attention to the ancient energy lines of the Urinary Bladder and Kidney meridians. Where our attention goes, our energy flows. I will practise asanas that stretch, squash, and squeeze along the Urinary Bladder and Kidney meridians.

> As I practise today, it is inclusive of all feelings, sensations, and circumstances as they arise. I will guide my attention with a gentle curiosity, an open heart, and kindness.

Beneficial Meditation

▷ Mindfulness of Body Practice, highlighting Kidney and Urinary Bladder meridians (chapter 7)
▷ Mindfulness of Emotions Practice / FEAR Practice (chapter 7)
▷ Gratitude practices (chapter 4)
▷ MBSM (chapter 7)

Practice Dedication

Finish by dedicating the value and virtue of your practice and sending kind thoughts.

For example:

> As I come the end this practice, I would like to dedicate its value and virtue and send some kind thoughts.

> As I breathe in, *May I be well and happy.* As I breathe out, *May [he, she, they] be well and happy.*

As you breathe in, allow your heart to fill with that intention and visualise yourself. As you breathe out, visualise an individual or a group of people and send that intention out to them. Practise this for three breaths.

Next, come to a comfortable seated position, bring your hands into a prayer position in front of your heart, and gently bow your head into anjali mudra. Take a moment to thank yourself for giving yourself the time and space to practise this morning, to attune to winter, and to fill your cup.

Bring your thumbs to your third eye centre as a gesture of honour, respect, and gratitude to yourself, to others, and to the practice experienced today.

Close with, "thank you/namaste."

Beneficial Water Element Sequence

Body tapping down BL & up KD meridians 3 times each, avoid if pregnant

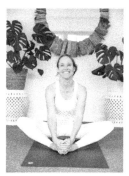

Butterfly plus set intention for practice whilst belly breathing & KD1 massage (3 minutes)

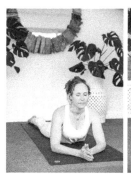

Sphinx (3-4 minutes), you can come up into Seal for the last minute if it is available to you

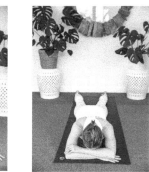

Prone Rebound (30-60 seconds)

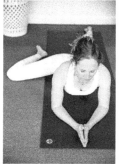

Half Frog/Half Lizard on left and then on right (1 minute each side)

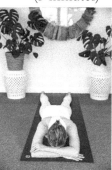

Prone Rebound (30-60 seconds)

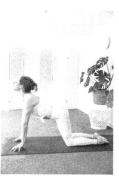

Cat/Cow (1 minute)

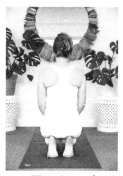

Toe Stretch (1-2 minutes)

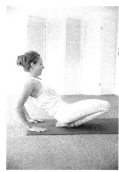

Ankle Stretch (1 minute)

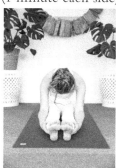

Caterpillar (3-4 minutes) then Seated Rebound

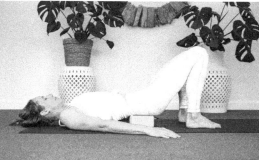 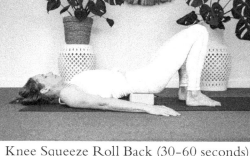

Knee Squeeze Roll Back (30-60 seconds) then Pelvic Lifts (1 minute) Supported Bridge (3-4 minutes) or One-Leg Supported Bridge on each side (2 mins each)

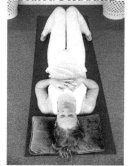

Rebound in CRP (30-60 seconds) then Knees to Chest

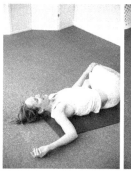 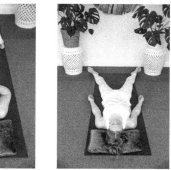

Reclining Twist or Twisted Roots each side (4 minutes each side including CRP in between sides)

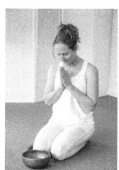

Savasana/CRP/ comfortable seat for chosen meditation

Seated Anjali Mudra plus dedication

Chapter 11
Spring

Spring is a time of growth and new beginnings. It is a time when we naturally feel like waking early with the rising sun and taking brisk invigorating walks outside. These are yang activities. Our energy and activity levels naturally start to increase in spring, and this flows into summer.

With an increase in rising energy comes an increase in creativity, determination, and strength. Plant life begins to sprout upwards following winter's slumber. The sight of tender young green plants and colourful blossoms nourishes our soul through the window of our eyes. Hence our appetite for food naturally decreases. Women can find it particularly beneficial and easier to practise intermittent fasting, do juice cleanses, or detox during this season. (Detailed information on intermittent fasting can be found in chapter 9, "Eat with the Seasons.")

Spring is naturally a time for cleansing, internally and externally. It is a time to cleanse ourselves of heavy food residues from winter and of any stagnant emotions and unhelpful habitual patterns. It's a time when we see things in new ways; a shift in perspective occurs. It's the season when we're naturally drawn towards external cleaning, such as clearing and cleaning our house. This is known as "spring cleaning." It's a time to take more care cleansing the outside of our body with dry skin brushing, face/body masks, and/or scrubs.

Spring corresponds to the wood element in TCM (the five element theory). The wood element involves our Liver and Gall Bladder meridians. It is believed these meridians are more vulnerable and prone to imbalance during spring and during the few weeks leading up to spring.

The main functions of the wood element are detoxification, maintaining even chi flow, and promotion of circulation and storage of the blood. As women, we need both a healthy supply and healthy circulation of blood at all times; this is even more the case during menstruation, pregnancy, labour, and breastfeeding. The Liver is very important in processing our hormones. As Joe Phee says, "Women need to prioritise care for their Liver."[1]

In addition to our Liver and Gall Bladder meridians being more susceptible to imbalance or blockage during spring, we also need to consider the everyday impact of our modern lifestyle. Artificial hormones, chemicals, medication, pollution, overconsumption of alcohol and caffeine, artificial colours, artificial flavours, preservatives, and unhealthy fats all disrupt Liver harmony. In our modern world the Liver is commonly the most congested and overworked of all the elemental organs.

The wood element is associated with the emotions of anger, frustration, irritability, and resentment. When we experience anger often, due to external circumstances, this can deplete and weaken the wood element. And vice versa, if our wood element is weak or imbalanced, then we will be more prone to anger and frustration. Mood swings and being "overly emotional" are all related to Liver imbalance. When our wood element is balanced, we feel kind and compassionate; we have an open perspective and are flexible and can adapt.

Those with balanced wood element:
- Have a calm and easy-going disposition
- Are kind and compassionate
- Are very organised
- Can make plans and put them into action
- Are flexible and able to change and adapt with ease
- Can be naturally effective leaders and decision-makers
- Are calm and composed in the face of change

> **Those with wood element imbalance may experience:**
> - Quickness to anger
> - Susceptibility to feeling frustrated, resentful, irritable, galled
> - Lack of motivation and indecisiveness
> - Eye problems (myopia at a young age)
> - Premenstrual symptoms, such as painful and irregular periods, flatulence, breast tenderness, breast cysts, and feeling overly emotional
> - Perimenopausal symptoms, like night sweats, cycle length changes, and rage
> - Allergies, hay fever, and headaches
> - Nerve pain, dizziness, muscle cramping, muscle weakness or stiffness, fatigue, arthritis, and types of paralysis
> - Poor circulation with cold hands and feet
> - Recurrent joint sprains and hypermobility

The poems, practices, and food suggestions in this chapter are to help support and nourish your wood element. This is important in the one to two weeks leading up to and during spring. The suggested asana sequence, pranayama and meditation practices are also helpful throughout the year if you are experiencing any of the aforementioned signs and symptoms of imbalance—in particular, if you are feeling premenstrual; hormonal; toxic (as a result of food, drink, chemicals, people, or the environment); or angry or have allergic rhinitis/hay fever.

Please note that a wood element nourishing asana sequence is generally more intense than the other elemental sequences because it focuses on stretching along the inner and outer thighs and hips. The hip and thigh areas commonly accumulate tension in the human body. Many of us store unprocessed emotions and tension in the hip region. Have you heard the saying, "We store issues in the tissues"?

Each time we experience a real or perceived threat, our sympathetic nervous system, our fight-flight response, is activated. We react by physically tensing the hip and thigh areas in readiness to fight or flee. Often, we do neither, fight nor flee, and instead we withdraw into ourselves. When we don't have the space, opportunity, or support to release this inner tension, it often accumulates in our hip area.

The space between our hips holds our second chakra, known as *Svadhisthana* in Sanskrit. Svadhisthana is associated with our emotional body, sensuality, intuition, and creativity. We can ignite svadhisthana by drawing our attention, with kindness and compassion, to our hips and the space between our hips and by performing hip opening poses. This opens us up to processing and understanding our emotions and to finding forgiveness. It can help us access our female intuition and our creativity.

If at any stage you feel overwhelmed during your asana and/or meditation practice, please redirect your attention to a more stable anchor. Feel your feet on the floor, take a deep belly breath, listen to sounds, and/or open your eyes.

Beneficial Food and Preparation

Aim to keep food preparation simple in spring. This is the time of year to have a light diet and avoid heavy, rich foods. Eat plenty of foods with upward energy such as young, above-ground plants, sprouts, fresh leafy greens, and lightly fermented foods.

Sprouting germinates grains, pulses, and seeds. This turns them into vitamin-rich, super-digestible baby plants. The sprouting process alters their protein structure, making the protein more digestible. It also alters the structure of any oligosaccharides and lectins, which again makes them more digestible. This results in less flatulence.

Avoid highly processed foods with preservatives, artificial flavours, and artificial colours. If there is a long list of unrecognisable ingredients and numbers on the packet, it is best to avoid the product. Simple, home-prepared meals are best all year round but particularly during spring.

Spring is a time when it is easier to eat less and lose weight. It is also the easiest time of year to fast, to internally cleanse your body, and to give your digestion a rest. (See the separate section on fasting in chapter 9, "Eat with the Seasons.")

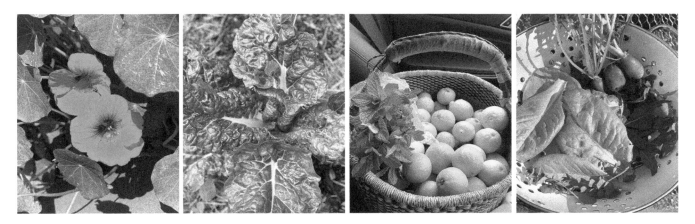

> **Victorian Spring Produce**
>
> Fruit—cumquat (end of citrus season), grapefruit, lemon, lime, mandarin, orange, strawberry (beginning of berry season)
>
> Herbs & Edible Flowers—bay leaf, basil, calendula, coriander, dahlia, lemon balm, mint, nasturtium, oregano, parsley, rosemary, sage, thyme
>
> Vegetables—asparagus, beetroot, broad bean, broccoli, cabbage, carrot, fennel, globe artichoke, leek, lettuce, pea, radish, rhubarb, rocket, silver beet/chard, spinach, spring onion
>
> Plentiful animal products—eggs, grass-fed lamb and beef

Wood Element Nourishment

Meridian Tapping and Acupressure

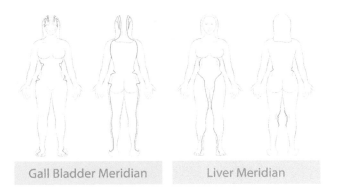

Gall Bladder Meridian Liver Meridian

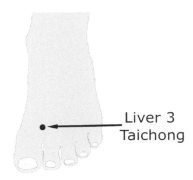

Liver 3
Taichong

Gall Bladder Meridian

The external Gall Bladder meridians begin at the outer corners of our eyes. From here they zigzag in front of the ears, behind the ears, along the sides of the head, down across the tops of the shoulders, around the front of the shoulders, and down either side of our torso. From the outer hips, they travel down along the outside of the legs, cross the outer ankles, and finish at the tip of our fourth toes.

Liver Meridian

The external Liver meridians begin at the inner edge of our big toenails. They then travel along the tops of our feet, past LV3, and up the inner leg; circle around our groin; and travel up the abdomen to finish at the lower chest at LV14.

LV3 Tai Chong / Great Rushing

These acupressure points are located at the top of the feet where the first and second toe tendons meet. When stimulated, they can help relieve chi stagnation. They are calming and are appropriately nicknamed the "cranky and irritable relieving spots"!

Wonder Full Poem and Quote

"My Version of the Serenity Prayer"
Grant us the serenity to accept the things we cannot change, the courage to change the things we can, and the wisdom, grace and gratitude to know the difference.

—Freya Bennett-Overstall

When we feel love and kindness towards others, it not only makes others feel loved and cared for, but it helps us also to develop inner happiness and peace.

—HHDL

"Spacious"

Dear you,
you who always have
so many things to do
so many places to be
your mind spinning like
fan blades at high speed
each moment always a blur
because you're never still

I know you're tired
I also know it's not your fault
The constant brain-buzz is like
a swarm of bees threatening
to sting if you close your eyes
You've forgotten something again
You need to prepare for that or else
You should have done that differently

What if you closed your eyes?
Would the world fall
apart without you?
Or would your mind
become the open sky
flock of thoughts
flying across the sunrise
as you just watched and smiled

—Kaveri Patel, *The Voice*[2]

Note: You can listen to Kaveri recite this poem on the Wisdom in Waves website, at https://www.wisdominwaves.com/about.html.

Intention for Practice

As you begin, please take a moment to pause and set your intention for practice today.

For example:

> I intend to cultivate mindful attention towards my body with its breath, my heart, and my mind during today's practice.

> I will nourish my wood element through certain mindful movement, pranayama, words, and meditation.

> I will pay particular attention to the ancient energy lines of the Liver and Gall Bladder meridians. Where our attention goes, our energy flows. I will practise asanas that stretch, squash, and squeeze along the Liver and Gall Bladder meridians.

> As I practise today, it is inclusive of all feelings, sensations, and circumstances as they arise. I will guide my attention with a gentle curiosity, an open heart, and kindness.

Beneficial Wood Element Meditation Practices

▷ Mindfulness of Body Practice highlighting liver and gall bladder meridians (chapter 7)
▷ Loving-Kindness (Metta/Maitri) (chapter 4)
▷ Mindfulness of Emotions Practice (chapter 7)
▷ MBSM (chapter 7)

Practice Dedication

Finish by dedicating the value and virtue of your practice and sending kind thoughts.

For example:

> As I come towards the end of this practice, I would like to dedicate its value and virtue and send some kind thoughts.

> As I breathe in, *May I be filled with loving-kindness.* As I breathe out, *May [he, she, they] be filled with loving-kindness.*

As you breathe in, allow your heart to fill with that intention and visualise yourself. As you breathe out, visualise an individual or a group of people and send that intention out to them. Practise this for three breaths.

Next come to a comfortable seated position, bring your hands into prayer position in front of your heart, and gently bow your head into anjali mudra. Take a moment to thank yourself for giving yourself the time and space to practise today, to attune to spring, and to fill your cup.

Bring your thumbs to your third eye centre as a gesture of honour, respect, and gratitude to yourself, to others, and to the practice experienced today.

Close with, "thank you/namaste."

Beneficial Wood Element Sequence

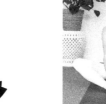

Body tapping down GB & up LV meridians 3 times each, skip if pregnant

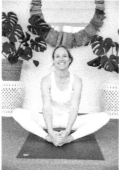

Butterfly plus set intention for practice whilst belly breathing & LV3 massage (3 minutes)

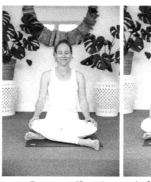

Square (3 minutes) followed by Seated Twist (2 minutes) followed by Windscreen Wipers (30–60 seconds), all done with right leg on top then repeat with left leg on top

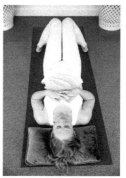

Rebound in CRP (30–60 seconds)

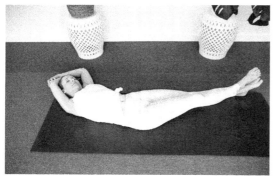

Bananasana stretch along right side and then along left side (3 minutes each side)

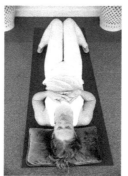

Rebound in CRP or hug knees to chest (30–60 seconds)

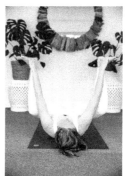

Happy Baby (3 minutes)

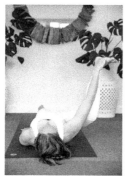 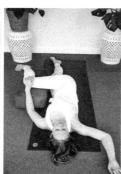 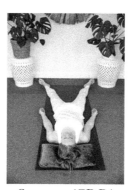

One-Leg Happy Baby (1 minute) then Reclining Twist (2 minutes) all with right leg, rebound in CRP, then repeat all with left leg

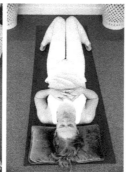

Savasana/CRP/ comfortable seat position for chosen meditation

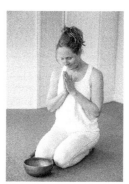

Seated Anjali Mudra plus seated dedication

Chapter 12
Summer

Summer is the season of abundance, when nature comes into maturity and life is in full bloom. We naturally awaken early on summer mornings and reach for the sun for nourishment, just as the plants and trees do. Have you ever planted a sunflower or watched a sunflower for a day? Its petals follow the sun.

Summer is the peak of yang. It's a time of light, warmth, and heat. Energy moves up and out with a lively brightness. As Paul Pitchford puts it, "The bounty of the outside world enters and enlivens us during summer."[1]

Summer corresponds to the fire element in TCM (the five element theory). There are four meridians involved in the fire element, and they are considered more vulnerable during this season—the Heart, Small Intestine, Pericardium, and Triple Heater meridians. The Triple Heater is also known as Triple Warmer or Triple Burner; all translations of *San Jiao*. In this book, we will focus on the two main fire meridians, the yin Heart meridian and the yang Small Intestine meridian.

The main functions of the fire element are governing our circulation, nervous system, memory, sleep, and our *shen*. Shen can be translated as our spirit, our consciousness, and/or our wakefulness. Our tender and brave heart is a haven for our shen, it is a place of wisdom and comfort. When our shen is sufficiently concentrated in the heart, our superficial thinking slows or stops. We become fully present with ease.

In TCM, your spirit, emotions, and consciousness all "reside" in the heart, which is why it's so important to work equally on your mind and body. We want to support our body with healthy exercise and food choices. However, it's just as important to support and strengthen our mind and mental health. Our mind has a big influence over our body's physical functioning. When our heart fire is not burning well, we are spiritless and have no zest for life.

The fire element is the most active, lively, and warming of the elements. When our fire element is out of balance, we experience the emotions of excessive joy, mania, hatred, and feeling muddled and lost. When our fire element is balanced, we experience natural joy, inner warmth, and peace.

Those with balanced fire element:
- Are happy, joyful, radiant
- Are genuinely friendly and have enthusiasm for life
- Have clarity
- Have heart-mind harmony
- Have the ability to give and receive love easily
- Sleep well
- Are humble due to perceiving the wonders of the world with their open heart

---

Those with fire element imbalance may experience:

- Poor blood circulation
- A ruddy or very pale complexion
- Weak spirit, spiritless
- Tiredness, fatigue, insomnia
- A scattered and confused mind, an overactive mind
- Being "burnt out"
- Feeling lost, vulnerable, extreme/excessive joy, frightfully overjoyed, manic, and/or depressed
- Excess or no laughter
- Palpitations, fast heartbeat
- Speech problems—stuttering, nonstop talking, confused speech
- Loss of memory
- Aversion to heat

The poems, practices, and food suggestions in this chapter are to help support and nourish your fire element. This is important in the one to two weeks leading up to and during summer. The suggested asana sequence, pranayama and meditation practices are also helpful throughout the year if you are experiencing any of the aforementioned signs and symptoms of imbalance.

Beneficial Summer Food and Preparation

Summer is a time of abundant food variety, so choose your meals to reflect this. Take advantage of all the different foods available during summer. Eat plenty of bright, colourful summer fruits and vegetables and enjoy creating beautiful-looking meals.

Cook lightly. Eat less. Eating heavy foods on hot days causes sluggishness. It can be helpful to lessen our meat, nut, and grain consumption on really hot days.

Limit overstimulating and hot spices during summer if you have a tendency towards anxiety and excess heat.

Red fruits and vegetables are said to nourish our fire element. So summer is the perfect time to enjoy all the delicious strawberries, raspberries, cherries, tomatoes, and red capsicum in season.

Foods with a bitter taste effect and nourish the fire element. Examples of bitter foods and herbs are cacao, chamomile, alfalfa sprouts, and romaine lettuce.

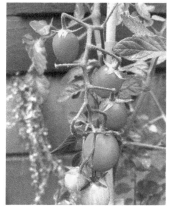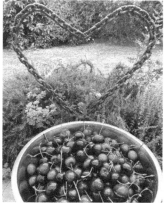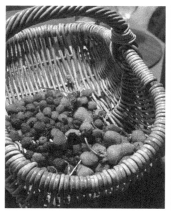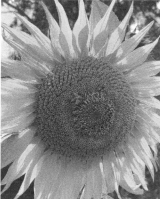

Fire Element Nourishment

Meridian Tapping and Acupressure

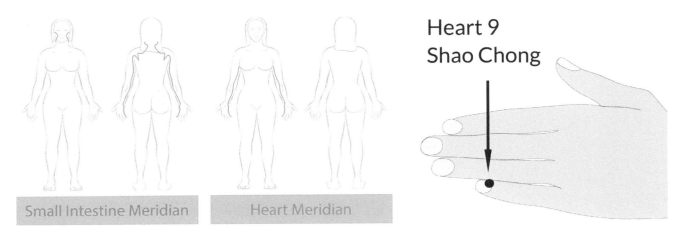

Small Intestine Meridian   Heart Meridian

Heart 9
Shao Chong

Heart Meridian

The Heart meridians originate internally in the heart and have three branches either side of the body. We will only explore the external Heart meridians, as this is where we tap. The external Heart meridians emerge from each armpit and run along the inner arms, ending at the inside tip of the little fingers where they connect with the Small Intestine meridians.

HT9 Shao Chong / Lesser Rushing

These acupressure points are located at the inner edge of the little fingernails. When stimulated they are said to calm the shen—balance the heart and mind. It is a very dynamic meeting point where the Heart meridians finish and the Small Intestine meridians start. We can gently massage these points during our practice using small circular movements and/or pulses, or we can apply direct pressure to these points.

Small Intestine Meridian

The external Small Intestine meridians start at the outside tip of the little fingers. They run upwards along the outside edge of the arms to the back of the shoulders. From the back of the shoulders, they travel up the sides of the neck and branch into two branches on each side of the head. One branch ends at the inner corner of the eyes and the other branch ends in the inner ears.

Wonder Full Poems and Quote

God help us to
Live slowly
To move simply
To look softly
To allow emptiness
To let the heart create for us
Amen.

—Michael Leunig[2]

When we close our heart, we cannot be joyful. When we have the courage to live with an open
heart, we are able to feel our pain and the pain of others, but we are also able to experience more
joy. The bigger and warmer our heart, the stronger our sense of aliveness and resilience.

—HHDL, *The Book of Joy*[3]

"Breath into Your Heart"
Breathe into your heart.
It knows the way.
It also knows when you must pause
and anchor into this moment,
when your body's hull is tossed
back and forth by thought waves
culminating into an emotional storm.

Breathe into your heart.
It is your wisest compass.
It knows when you are ready
to travel again towards True North,
the direction of non-harming,
when you can be a guiding light
for other ships lost at sea.

—Kaveri Patel, *Awakening*[4]

Intention for Fire Element Nourishing Practice

As you begin, please take a moment to pause and set your intention for your practice today.
For example:

I intend to cultivate mindful attention towards my body with its breath, my heart, and my mind during today's practice.

I will nourish my fire element through certain movement, words, and meditation.

I will pay particular attention to the ancient energy lines of the Heart and Small Intestine meridians. Where our attention goes, our energy flows. I will practise asanas that stretch, squash, and squeeze along the Heart and Small Intestine meridians.

I will open my brave and tender heart as best I can during today's practice. My heart is full of wisdom and compassion.

As I practise today, it is inclusive of all feelings, sensations, and circumstances as they arise. I will guide my attention with a gentle curiosity, an open heart, and kindness.

Beneficial Fire Element Meditation Practices

▷ Mindfulness of Body Practice highlighting Heart and Small Intestine meridians (chapter 7)
▷ A loving-kindness meditation (Maitri/Metta) (chapter 4)
▷ MBSM (chapter 7)

Practice Dedication

Finish by dedicating the value and virtue of your practice and sending kind thoughts.

For example:

As I come towards the end of this practice, I would like to dedicate its value and virtue and send some kind thoughts.

As I breathe in, *May I be filled with loving-kindness.* As I breathe out, *May [he, she, they] be filled with loving-kindness.*

As you breathe in, allow your heart to fill with this intention and visualise yourself. As you breathe out, visualise an individual or a group of people and send that intention out to them. Practise this for three breaths.

Next, come to a comfortable seated position, bring your hands into a prayer position in front of your heart, and gently bow your head into anjali mudra. Take a moment to thank yourself for giving yourself the time and space to practise today, to attune to summer, and to fill your cup.

Bring your thumbs to your third eye centre as a gesture of honour, respect, and gratitude to yourself, to others, and to the practice experienced today.

Close with, "thank you/namaste."

Beneficial Fire Element Sequence

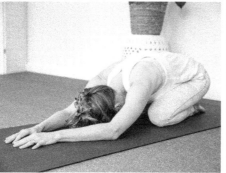 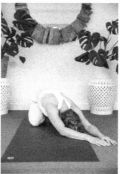 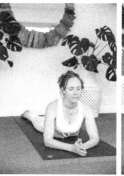

Body tapping down HT & up SI meridians 3 times each, skip if pregnant

Child's Pose with arms out long in front plus long exhale breath as you set your intention for practice & press little fingers down into mat, stimulating HT9 (3 minutes)

Child's Pose with side stretch to left and then to right (1 minute each side)

Sphinx, (3-4 minutes), you can come up into Seal for the last minute if it is available to you

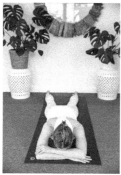 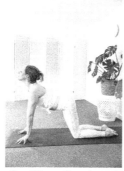 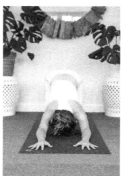

Prone Rebound (1 minute)

Cat/Cow (1 minute)

Melting Heart (3 minutes) or Half Melting Heart left then right (90 seconds each arm)

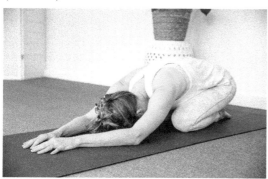 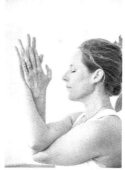 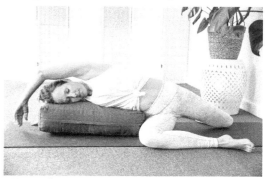

Seated Rebound or Child's Pose (1 minute)

Eagle Arms each side (1 minute each arm)

Twisted Deer with right arm above (3 minutes) Windscreen Wipers then swap sides to Twisted Deer with left arm above (3 minutes)

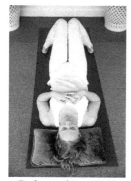 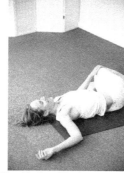 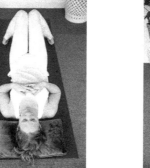 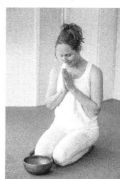

Rebound in CRP (30-60 seconds) then Knees to Chest

Reclining Twist or Twisted Roots each side (4 minutes each side including CRP in between sides)

Savasana/CRP/ comfortable seat for chosen meditation

Seated Anjali Mudra plus dedication

Chapter 13
Late Summer

Late summer is a short and relatively unrecognised season. It's approximately the last month of summer. It's the transition point between the expansive yang of the spring and summer months, and the inward yin of the autumn and winter months. It's a time for us to prepare and nourish ourselves for the inward cooling yin seasons to come.

This fifth season corresponds to the earth element in TCM (five element theory). The earth element involves our Spleen and Stomach meridians. These meridians are believed to be more vulnerable during late summer.

Our Spleen and Stomach meridians are primarily responsible for digestion, nourishment, and metabolism. Our diet and eating habits heavily impact these meridians.

Major causes of weak earth element and digestive troubles are:
- Eating too quickly
- Eating when stressed
- Overeating
- Overconsumption of rich and greasy foods
- Too many cold drinks/ice creams
- Too many sweets/high sugar food
- Irregular eating
- Overconsumption of cold foods and raw vegetables
- Microbiome imbalance

The earth element is associated with the emotions of worry, anxiety, low self-esteem, and over sympathy. When we regularly experience these emotions, this can deplete the earth element. And vice versa, if someone has a weak or imbalanced earth element, then the person will be more prone to experiencing these emotions. People who have a balanced earth element feel grounded, at ease, creative and have a healthy self-esteem.

Those with a balanced earth element:
- Nurture themselves and others
- Are generally hard-working, practical, and responsible
- Are strong and active with good muscle tone
- Are creative and clear thinking
- Have a good appetite and digestion
- Feel trust, openness, and positive self-esteem
- Are grounded, balanced, and content
- Find that their various body cycles are in harmony; these include sleep cycles, breath, thinking, and menstruation

---

The poems, practices, pranayama, and food suggestions in this chapter are all to help support and nourish your earth element. This is important during late summer and the few weeks leading up to it. The suggested asana sequence, pranayama and meditation practices are also helpful throughout the year if you are experiencing any of the aforementioned signs and symptoms of imbalance.

Spending time in nature harmonises your earth element. So does exercise, getting enough sleep, regular meditation, and "me" time. Centring breath practices are very helpful too.

During the earth element nourishing asana sequence, we focus on backbends and lunges, which stretch along the Stomach and Spleen meridians.

Beneficial Foods

It's best to keep meals simple with minimal seasoning and a small number of ingredients during late summer. Choose to eat more warming meals over cold dishes. Lightly cook your food.

Naturally sweet foods build and strengthen the earth element and, ultimately, the entire body. Remember we need a balance though, not too much sweet, which is easily done with refined lollies, soft drinks, and baked goods.

Foods that are yellow and golden in colour also nourish the earth element. Round foods, such as cabbage, peaches, and millet are considered harmonising and helpful during late summer.

We can benefit our earth element by eating slowly and chewing our food thoroughly. This not only helps break down and digest the food, but it also gives your brain a chance to catch up with your stomach, so that you will know when you are full.

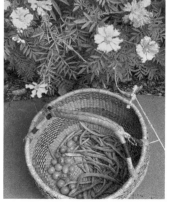
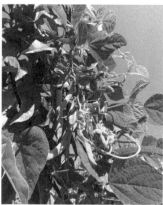
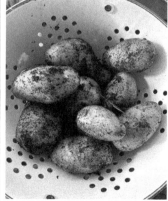
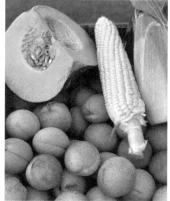

Earth Element Nourishment

Meridian Tapping and Acupressure

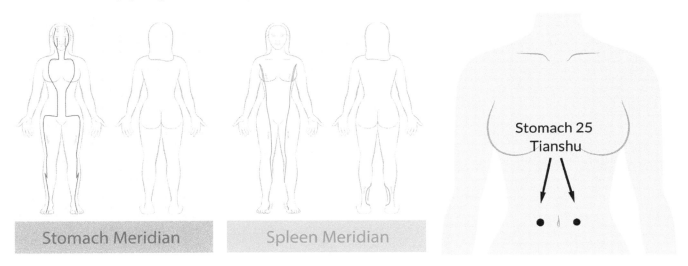

Stomach Meridian

The external Stomach meridians start just under the eyes. They run down the centre of the face, curve towards the bridge of the nose and then around the mouth. From the lower jaw they run down the neck to the sternum, down the front of the body passing through the nipples, down the front of the legs and finish at the tip of the second toes.

ST 25 Tianshu / Celestial Pivot

These acupressure points lie three finger widths either side of the midline, in line with the navel. When stimulated, they are said to help digestive issues such as constipation, diarrhea, bloating, and pain. They also help menstrual irregularities, menstrual pain, fibroids, ovarian cysts, and fluid retention. We can gently massage these points during our earth element practice.

Spleen Meridian

The external Spleen meridians start at the tip of the big toes. They then run along the inner feet, up the inner legs, across the sides of the groin, and up the outer sides of the torso and finish in the armpits.

Wonder Full Poem and Quote

"I Worried"
I worried a lot. Will the garden grow, will the rivers
flow in the right direction, will the earth turn
as it was taught, and if not, how shall
I correct it?

Was I right, was I wrong, will I be forgiven,
can I do better?

Will I ever be able to sing, even the sparrows
can do it and I am, well,
hopeless.

Is my eyesight fading or am I just imagining it,
am I going to get rheumatism,
lockjaw, dementia?

Finally I saw that worrying had come to nothing.
And I gave it up. And I took my old body
and went out into the morning
and sang.
—Mary Oliver, *Swan: Poems and Prose Poems*[1]

Intention for Earth Element Nourishing Practice

As you begin, please take a moment to pause and set your intention for practice today.
For example:

I intend to cultivate mindful attention towards my body with its breath, my heart, and my mind during today's practice.

I will nourish my earth element through certain asanas, words, and meditation.

I will pay particular attention to the ancient energy lines of the Stomach and Spleen meridians. Where our attention goes, our energy flows. I will practise asanas that stretch, squash, and squeeze along the Stomach and Spleen meridians. I will also focus on deep belly breaths, which help with centring and grounding. I acknowledge this is particularly important during late summer.

As I practise today, it is inclusive of all feelings, sensations, and circumstances as they arise. I will guide my attention with a gentle curiosity, an open heart, and kindness.

Beneficial Meditation

▷ Mindfulness of Breath Practice (chapter 7)
▷ Mindfulness of Body Practice highlighting Stomach and Spleen meridians (chapter 7)
▷ Full MBSM (chapter 7)

Practice Dedication

Finish by dedicating the value and virtue of the practice and sending kind thoughts.

For example:

> As I come towards the end of this practice, I would like to dedicate its value and virtue and send some kind thoughts.

> As I breathe in, *May I be peaceful and at ease.* As I breathe out, *May [he,she,they] be peaceful and at ease.*

As you breathe in, allow your heart to fill with that intention and visualise yourself. As you breathe out, visualise an individual or a group of people and send that intention out to them. Practise this for three breaths.

Next, come to a comfortable seated position, bring your hands into prayer position in front of your heart, and gently bow your head into anjali mudra. Take a moment to thank yourself for giving yourself the time and space to practise this morning, to attune to late summer, and to fill your cup.

Bring your thumbs to your third eye centre as a gesture of honour, respect, and gratitude to yourself, to others and to the practice experienced today.

Close with, "thank you/namaste."

Beneficial Earth Element Sequence

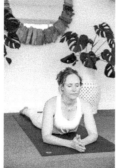

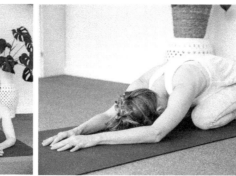

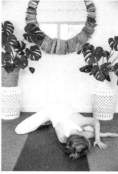

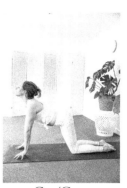

Body tapping down the ST & up the SP meridians 3 times each, skip if pregnant

Sphinx plus long exhalation breath as you set your intention for your practice (3 minutes)

Child's Pose plus long exhalation breath (3 minutes)

Wide Child's Pose with Twist to right side then left (3 minutes each side) with seated rebound

Cat/Cow (1 minute)

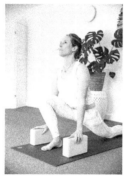

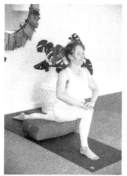

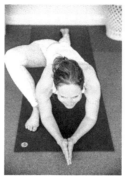

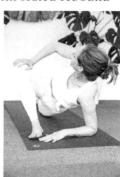

Dragon series on right side then left side (5 minutes in total each side); spend 1 minute in each– Tennis Ball Dragon, High Dragon, Low Dragon, then Twisted Dragon; slow release & rebound by shifting your weight backwards & straightening out your front leg which offers a hamstring stretch

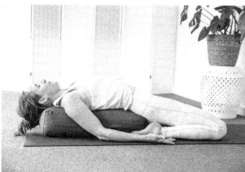

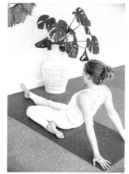

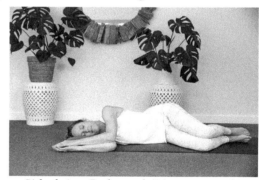

Supported Saddle (4 minutes) or Half Saddle (2 minutes each side) with ST25 massage

Side-lying Rebound (30–60 seconds)

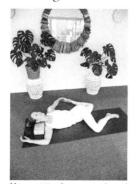

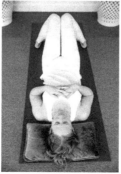

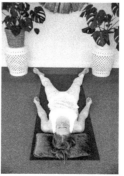

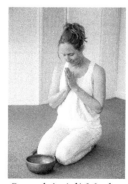

Cat Pulling Tail on right then left (3 minutes each side) with Side-lying Rebound in between sides

Side-lying/CRP/ Savasana rebound (1 minute)

Savasana/CRP/comfortable seated position for chosen meditation

Seated Anjali Mudra plus dedication

Chapter 14
A Little Extra

Supportive Wall Practice

The following wall sequence is wonderfully restorative. It offers a super-duper dose of self-care. It can be practised any time of the year. It's helpful if you're feeling exhausted, have been on your feet all day, or have been for a long run or ride. It also helps with fluid retention in the legs (from heat, a long-haul flight, or lymphatic insufficiency) and restless legs.

Wonder Full Photo and Quote

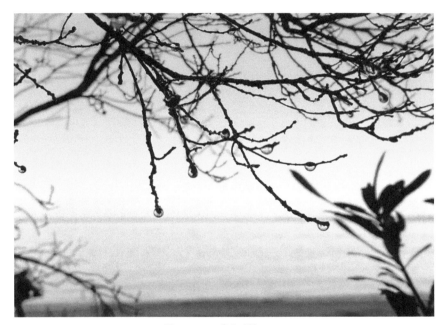

Drops of Stillness

Indigenous elder Miriam-Rose Ungunmerr was awarded Senior Australian of the Year in early 2021. This was in recognition of her role as a teacher, an artist, and a role model in her community and for her introduction of *dadirri* to the world.

"*Dadirri* is a reflection written by Miriam-Rose Ungunmerr from the Nauiyu Community, Daly River, Northern Territory. The word, concept, and spiritual practice that is *dadirri* (da-did-ee) is from the Ngan'gikurunggurr and Ngen'giwumirri languages of the Aboriginal peoples of the Daly River region (Northern Territory, Australia)"[1].

Dadirri involves inner, deep listening and quiet, still awareness.

Dadirri recognises the deep spring that is inside us. We call on it and it calls to us. This is the gift that Australia is thirsting for. It is something like what you call contemplation.

When I experience dadirri, I am made whole again. I can sit on the riverbank or walk through the trees; even if someone close to me has passed away, I can find my peace in this silent awareness. There is no need of words. A big part of dadirri is listening.

...

The contemplative way of dadirri spreads over our whole life. It renews us and brings us peace. It makes us feel whole again.

And now I would like to talk about the other part of dadirri which is the quiet stillness and the waiting.

Our Aboriginal culture has taught us to be still and to wait. We do not try to hurry things up. We let them follow their natural course—like the seasons. We watch the moon in each of its phases. We wait for the rain to fill our rivers and water the thirsty earth.

When twilight comes, we prepare for the night. At dawn we rise with the sun.

We watch the bush foods and wait for them to ripen before we gather them. We wait for our young people as they grow, stage by stage, through their initiation ceremonies. When a relation dies, we wait a long time with the sorrow. We own our grief and allow it to heal slowly.

—Miriam-Rose[2]

I encourage you to read Miriam-Rose's full reflection on dadirri, which can be found on the Miriam-Rose Foundation website. The Foundation uses the four pillars of art, culture, education, and opportunity to help young indigenous people walk in the two worlds of modern Australia and indigenous Australia. The website can be found at https://www.miriamrosefoundation.org.au/.

Intention for Practice

As you begin, please take a moment to pause and set your intention for practice today.
For example:

I intend to cultivate mindful attention towards my body with its breath, my heart, and my mind during today's practice.

Let wonderful drops of dadirri fall softy through my practice today.

As I practise today, it is inclusive of all feelings, sensations, and circumstances as they arise. I will guide my attention with a gentle curiosity, an open heart, and kindness.

Practice Dedication

Finish by dedicating the value and virtue of your practice and sending kind thoughts:

As I come towards the end of this practice, I would like to dedicate its value and virtue and send some kind thoughts.

As I breathe in, *May I be well and happy.* As I breathe out, *May [he, she, they] be well and happy.*
As you breathe in, allow your heart to fill with that intention and visualise yourself. As you breathe out, visualise an individual or a group of people and send that intention out to them. Practise this for three breaths.
Next, come to a comfortable seated position, bring your hands into a prayer position in front of your heart, and gently bow your head into anjali mudra. Take a moment to thank yourself for giving yourself the time and space to practise this morning, to allow for moments of dadirri, and to fill your cup.
Bring your thumbs to your third eye centre as a gesture of honour, respect, and gratitude to yourself, to others, and to the practice experienced today.
Close with, "thank you/namaste."

Beneficial Wall Sequence

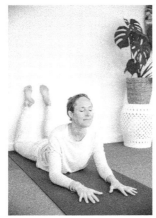

Wall Sphinx plus set your intention for practice whilst deep belly breathing (3-4 minutes)

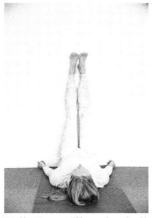

Wall Caterpillar plus belly breath (3-4 minutes)

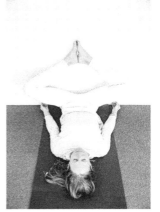

Wall Butterfly (3-4 minutes)

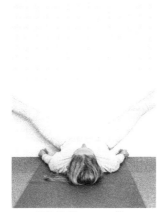

Wall Dragonfly (3-4 minutes)

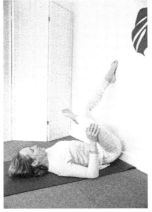

Wall Eye of Needle with right leg and then left leg (3-4 minutes each side) plus massage your masseter (jaw muscle) on same side as hip stretch for first minute

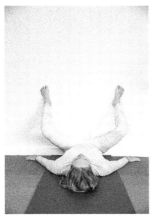

Wall Squat plus belly breath (3-4 minutes)

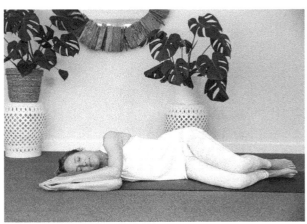

Right Side-lying Rebound (30-60 seconds)

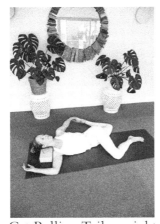

Cat Pulling Tail on right then left (3 minutes each side) with Side-lying Rebound in between sides

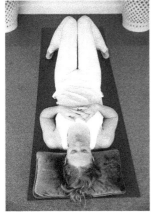

Side-lying/CRP/Savasana rebound (1 minute)

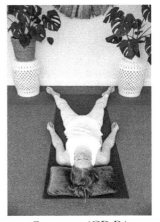

Savasana/CRP/ comfortable seated position for chosen meditation

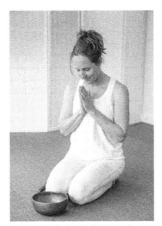

Seated Anjali Mudra plus dedication

My Chocolate Hazelnut Spread Recipe

Ingredients

- 125g of locally grown roasted hazelnuts
- 100g of good quality, ethically sourced dark chocolate
- 40g of locally grown and produced mild-tasting olive oil

Method

▷ Whiz the hazelnuts into a paste with Thermomix (TMX) on speed 9.
▷ Scrape down the sides of the TMX bowl and add in the chocolate, broken into chunks. Set TMX to 70C, speed 6, five minutes or until chocolate is melted.
▷ Scrape down the sides of the TMX bowl again and add olive oil. Whiz up to TMX speed 9.
▷ Scrape down the sides of TMX bowl again and pour into a clean jar, keep in the fridge. It won't last long.

I like to spread it onto homemade Life-Changing Gluten Free Sourdough Crumpets[3] and sprinkle fresh pomegranate seeds, slices of fresh strawberries, blueberries, or cherries on top (depending on what fruit is in season).

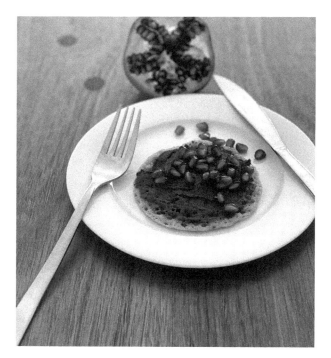

Appendix A
List of Abbreviations

AK. applied kinesiology

BL. bladder meridian

CRP. constructive rest pose

GB. gall bladder meridian

HHDL. His Holiness the Dalai Lama

HT. heart meridian

KD. kidney meridian

LV. liver meridian

LI. large intestine meridian

LU. lung meridian

NET. neuro emotional technique

MBSM. mindfulness-based stillness meditation

PC. pericardium meridian

PNS. parasympathetic nervous system

SI. small intestine meridian

SP. spleen meridian

ST. stomach meridian

SNS. sympathetic nervous system

TCM. traditional Chinese medicine

TH. triple heater / triple warmer / triple burner / San Jiao meridian

Appendix B
Sanskrit Words Commonly Used

asana. Pose.

anjali mudra. Refers to the hand position with palms resting in a prayer position in front of the heart with the head slightly bowed.

mula bandha. Root lock. This is activated by contracting the pelvic floor and drawing upwards towards the spine.

namaste. I bow to you.

pranayama. The practice of focusing on and altering our breath.

savasana. Corpse pose. Lie on your back, legs slightly apart, palms open resting by your side or on your belly.

svadhyaya. Self-inquiry, self-study.

ujjayi breath. Victorious breath. It involves the long slow breaths with a slight constriction at the back of the throat that activate our parasympathetic nervous system.

Seasonal Practice Summary Table

Season	Spring	Summer	Late Summer	Autumn	Winter
Element	Wood	Fire	Earth	Metal	Water
Environmental Influence	Wind	Heat	Damp	Dry	Cold
Development	Birth	Growth	Transformation	Harvest	Storage
Colour	Green	Red	Yellow	White	Black/dark blue
Beneficial Foods Eat what is in season in your local area.	Eat less, or even fast, to cleanse the body. Your diet should be the lightest of the year; avoid heavy foods. Eat young plants, sprouts, and fresh *greens*. Include lightly fermented food. Drink fresh mint and peppermint tea/infusions.	Eat light foods and some raw foods. Eat large leafy greens, summer squashes, fruit in season and, *red* food—tomatoes, cherries, raspberries, strawberries, capsicum. Include lighter grains such as white long-grain rice (basmati in particular) and barley.	Eat mildly sweet foods and *yellow* or *golden*-coloured foods—sweet corn, sweet potato, carrots, pumpkin, cantaloupe, peaches, apricots. Eat round, grounding foods—cabbage, soybeans, millet. Include rice, sweet rice, and amaranth.	Eat foods of concentrated quality—slow cooking will do this—and add warm and pungent spices. Eat root vegetables, winter squash, beans, and *white* foods—cabbage, radish, cauliflower, onion, garlic. Include grains such as sweet rice, mochi, and millet.	Eat foods of concentrated quality. Royal jelly and bee pollen, micro-algae (chlorella, spirulina, wild-blue algae), and organic organ meats are all strengthening foods. To tonify Kidney chi eat beans and black/dark-coloured food—black sesame, black beans, black seaweed, black fungus, black soybeans. Include chestnuts, walnuts, almonds, high-quality milk, nettles, salty foods. Include heavier grains such as sweet rice, buckwheat, and oats.
Beneficial Food Preparation	Simple food preparation of raw, light steaming, pressing, pickling, and sprouting.	Create beautiful meals. Simple preparation of raw, blanching, light steaming, quick sauté, and simmer. Use a little salt and more water.	Keep meals simple. Cook lightly with moderate steaming, low heat cooking, and boiling. Minimal seasoning and mild taste	More focused food preparation by sautéing and then covered simmering, baking, soups, and slow cooked stews. Cook with less water and at lower heat for longer.	More focused food preparation by stewing, frying, soups, stews, and crockery cooking/slow cooker. Cook foods longer, at lower temperatures, and with less water.

Beneficial Flavour	Sour Adjusts Wood	Bitter Adjusts Fire	Sweet Adjusts Earth	Spicy (Pungent) Adjusts Metal	Salty Adjusts Water
Yin Organ	Liver	Heart	Spleen	Lung	Kidney
Yang Organ	Gall Bladder	Small Intestine	Stomach	Large Intestine	Urinary Bladder
Tissue	Tendons and ligaments	Blood vessels	Muscles	Skin and hair	Bone and teeth
Sense Organ	Eyes-sight	Tongue-speech	Tongue-taste	Nose-smell	Ear-hearing
Functions	Detoxification, blood storage, promotion of circulation, and emotional regulation	Circulation, shen (consciousness), sleep, nervous system regulation, memory, and love	Digestion, distribution of food and nutrients, and metabolism	Immunity, respiration (expiration), nourishment, vocal expression, and balance of moisture in the body	Water metabolism, longevity, bone strength (including teeth), reproduction, physical and mental maturation
Emotions	Anger, resentment, aggression, frustration, irrationality, stubborn	Lost, vulnerable, muddled, frightfully overjoyed, manic	Worry, anxiety, over sympathetic, over concern, low self-esteem	Grief, sadness, yearning, dogmatically positioned, defensive, melancholy	Fear, dread, paralysed will, inefficient
Balanced Characteristics	Kind, receptive	Loving, joyful	Creative, grounded, good self-esteem	Aware of beauty, wonder and awe	Wise, mature
Meditation Emphasis	Mindfulness of Body highlighting Liver and Gall Bladder meridians, Loving-kindness, Mindfulness of Emotions, MBSM	Mindfulness of Body highlighting Heart and Small Intestine meridians, Loving-kindness, MBSM	Mindfulness of Body highlighting Spleen and Stomach meridians, Mindfulness of Breath, MBSM	Mindfulness of Body highlighting Lung and Large Intestine meridians, Mindfulness of Breath, Mindfulness of Emotions, gratitude, MBSM	Mindfulness of Body highlighting Kidney and Urinary Bladder meridians, Mindfulness of Emotions, FEAR Practice, gratitude, MBSM
Common Resistance	Busy thoughts, restlessness, boredom, agitation, impatience	Busy thoughts, restlessness, boredom, agitation, impatience	Busy thoughts, restlessness, boredom, agitation, impatience	Dull mind, sleepiness	Dull mind, sleepiness

Acknowledgement and Gratitude

Most of this book was dreamt, drawn, and written on Boon Wurrung Country of the Kulin Nation. I acknowledge and graciously thank the traditional custodians, past, present, and emerging of this precious Country.

This book has been written with the support and encouragement of many people in my life.

First, my invaluable friend, first reader, and born editor Tania Kennelly, this book would not be here without you; thank you. And a big thank you also goes to your kids, Amelia, Max, and James for all their support and input.

Thank you to all the participants of my classes, workshops, and retreats. You are my inspiration to write this book. A special thanks to Ana, Brig, Fipe, Marg, Nina, and Val for your support and for allowing me to share your stories. Michelle and Fleur, thank you for being book-sounding boards in the early days; your encouragement to continue lifted my heart and made writing easier. A further thanks to Ana for all your support with opening Maitri Studio Brighton, along with retreats and workshops. You bless each space with your creative kokedamas, love, and intuition.

Heartfelt thanks go to Simone Davis, Lucas Collins, Verity Scott, Lucas Overstall, and Zachary Overstall for inviting and supporting me to teach mindfulness at Caulfield Grammar School and Scotch College. This came about due to our eldest son, Lucas, asking me to share mindfulness at school (when he was in year three) and telling his then teacher, Simone Davis, about me.

Thank you to my mum, Sally, for introducing me to yoga and Buddhism at such a young age. And thank you for providing me with the opportunity to meet HHDL when I was seventeen. He left a powerful impression of overflowing compassion, humility, and wonder.

Many thanks and the squashiest of squeezes go to my "little sister" Cassia for her support and encouragement and for being my first ever and longest running "student."

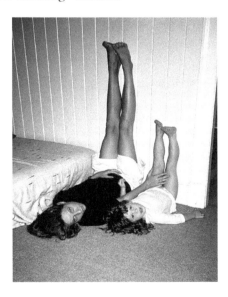

My love of plants, nature and home-grown goodies started early, with direction from my dad and stepmum, Nigel and Pip. This was further encouraged by my inspirational green-thumbed grandmother, Edith. Many thanks go to the three of you.

Zo, thank you for always supporting and encouraging me to create—be that through my writing, walking around your garden, weaving together, shibori dyeing together, sharing cooking and recipes, or pottery and natural printing together. The list goes on.

Caroline, I have you to thank for encouraging my love of dance and respect for our bodies and introducing me to chiropractic—and so much more.

Vicki Anthonisz, thank you for your continuing encouragement, love, belief and regular chiropractic and NET adjustments. You are an angel.

Nick Conquest, thank you for all our TCM discussions and your support, both in writing this book and with my health.

Georgie, we have always shared a love of books. Your recommendation of the podcast *The Secret Life of Writers* has been a book saver. Each time fear and doubt started to build, I would listen to one of the podcast episodes and be able to continue writing. Plus, you inspired me by writing your own book; this provided me with the extra nudge I needed to start writing myself.

Corinne, I offer heartfelt thanks to you for giving me the kind and gentle nudge to return to yoga, namely, to try yin yoga, when I thought I physically couldn't do yoga asana anymore.

Ali Mayfield, thank you for helping me relax in front of the camera whilst you worked your magic and for all your patience and expertise readying photos for print in this book.

Many thanks to Karen Bravo for helping me bring my Seasonal Woman illustration to life in the digital realm. All of your creative work with the feminine form is so colourful, fertile, and fluid.

Many thanks go to all the teachers I have been blessed with, particularly my children, Lucas and Zac, as well as Bob Sharples, Bernie Clark, Dustin Brown, HHDL, Janet Etty-Leal, Jo Phee, Paul Bedson, Pema Chodron, Sarah Powers, Thupten Jinpa, and Thupten Lekshe.

Simon, "Spunky," thank you for allowing me the space to write this book. And thank you for being a sounding board about the process, particularly as you have already written two books yourself and (I've lost count how) many scientific papers.

I am so grateful for all the wonderful women and marvellous men in my life who I have the privilege to call friends. You all have a part to play in my writing of this book. Thank you.

And lastly, many thanks go to the publishing team at Balboa Press and Hay House for helping me release this book into the world, with a special thanks to Jad for his patience and support.

Bibliography

Apsrey, Dave. *Fast This Way: Burn Fat, Heal Inflammation, and Eat Like the High-Performing Human You Were Meant to Be*. London, UK: Harper Collins Publishers, 2021.

Caruthers, Cara. *Eat Like You Love Yourself: A Modern Guide to Ayurvedic Cooking and Living*. Australia: Self Published, 2018.

Clark, Bernie. *The Complete Guide to Yin Yoga: The Philosophy and Practice of Yin Yoga*. 1st ed. Vancouver, BC, Canada: Wild Strawberry Productions, 2018.

Gawler, Ian, and Paul Bedson, Paul. *Meditation: An In-Depth Guide*. Sydney, Australia: Allen & Unwin Publishers, 2010.

Hill, Maisie. *Period Power*. London: Green Tree, Bloomsbury Publishing, 2019.

Hill, Maisie. *Perimenopause Power*. London: Green Tree, Bloomsbury Publishing. 2021.

His Holiness the Dalai Lama, Archbishop Desmond Tutu, and Douglas Abrams. *The Book of Joy: Lasting Happiness in a Changing World*. London, UK: Penguin Random House UK, 2016.

Isaacs, Jennifer, ed. *Australian Dreaming: 40,000 Year of Aboriginal History*. Sydney, Australia: New Holland Publishers, 2005.

Kimmerer, Robin Wall. *Braiding Sweetgrass: Indigenous Wisdom, Scientific Knowledge, and the Teachings of Plants*. London, UK: Penguin UK, 2020.

Lama Zopa Rinpoche. *Ultimate Healing: The Power of Compassion*. Somerville, MA, USA: Wisdom Publications, 2001.

Lyttleton, Jane. *Treatment of Infertility with Chinese Medicine*. 2nd ed. Edinburgh: Churchill Livingstone Elsevier, 2013.

Napthali, Sarah. *Buddhism for Mothers with Lingering Questions*. Sydney, Australia: Inspired Living, 2007.

Myers, Thomas W. *Anatomy Trains: Myofascial Meridians for Manual Therapists and Movement Therapists*. 4th ed. China: Elsevier Limited, 2021.

Oliver, Mary. *New And Select Poems*. Vol. 2. Boston: Beacon Press, 2005.

Patel, Kaveri. *The Voice*. Self-published, 2014.

Patel, Kaveri. Awakening. Self-published, 2021.

Pitchford, Paul. *Healing with Whole Foods: Asian Traditions and Modern Nutrition*. 3rd ed. Berkeley: North Atlantic Books, 2002.

Porges, Stephen. *The Polyvagal Theory: Neurophysiological Foundations of Emotions, Attachment, Communication, and Self-Regulation*. W.W. Norton & Company, Inc., 2011.

Powers, Sarah. *Insight Yoga*. Boulder: Shambala Publications, 2008.

Professor Lun Wong and Kath Knapsey. *Food for the Seasons: Eat Well and Stay Healthy the Traditional Chinese Way.* Melbourne: Red Dog, 2002.

Purbrick, Matt, and Lentil. *Grown and Gathered: Traditional Living Made Modern.* Sydney: Pan Macmillan, 2016.

Reid, Daniel. *The Tao of Health, Sex, and Longevity: A Modern, Practical Approach to the Ancient Way.* London: Simon and Schuster, 1989.

Rumi. *The Essential Rumi.* Translated by Coleman Barks. New York: Harper One, Harper Collins Publishers, 2004.

Sharples, Bob. *Meditation: Calming the Mind.* South Melbourne: Lothian, 2003.

Thich Nhat Hanh. *Old Path White Clouds: Walking in the Footsteps of the Buddha.* 19th Ed. New Delhi: Full Circle Publishing, 2015.

Thich Nhat Hanh, *The Miracle of Mindfulness.* London: Rider, 2008.

Yunkaporta, Tyson. *Sand Talk: How Indigenous Thinking Can Save the World.* Melbourne: Text Publishing Company, 2019.

Villoldo, Alberto, Dr. *Grow a New Body: How Spirit and Power Plant Nutrients Can Transform Your Health.* Carlsbad, California: Hay House Inc, 2019.

Resources

Useful Apps Mentioned:
- Insight Timer
- Period Diary
- What's Good

Wonderful Websites:

https://www.compassioninstitute.com/

    The Compassion Institute advocates for and provides compassion education globally.

https://www.dalailama.com/

https://feetup.com/

    You can find further information here on inversions with the FeetUp Trainer.

https://www.freyabennettoverstall.com/

    Video recordings of classes and seasonal practices, guided meditation recording links, blog, poems, and class bookings.

https://www.futurefoodsystem.com/

    An inspirational self-sustaining zero waste house. Imagine solving the world's biggest problems simply by changing the way we live.

https://www.grownandgathered.com.au/

    Growing food, gathering, and sharing with the seasons.

https://insighttimer.com/

    The number one free app for sleep, anxiety, and stress. You will find many of my guided recordings available here.

https://www.lowtoxlife.com/

    Valuable information, podcasts, courses, and resources on how to live a low-tox life.

https://www.maisiehill.com/

    Are you ready to harness your hormones and get your cycle working for you?

https://www.1millionwomen.com.au/

https://www.miriamrosefoundation.org.au/

    Empowering indigenous futures through art, cultures, education, and opportunity.

https://museumsvictoria.com.au/melbournemuseum/resources/forest-secrets/

    The eastern Kulin Nation seasonal calendar and further information can be sourced here.

https://pipmagazine.com.au/

> Nourish yourself and the planet with ideas and inspiration for a positive future, delivered to your door and on your devices.

https://sarahpowersinsightyoga.com/teachings/

https://www.soundstrue.com/

> Sounds true offers transformational programs to help you live a more genuine, loving, and meaningful life.

https://terrywahls.com/

> Dr Terry Wahls' research-backed strategies for managing multiple sclerosis and other autoimmune diseases.

https://www.wisdominwaves.com/about.html

> Kaveri Patel's website filled with her wonderful poems and some recordings of her guided meditations.

https://yinspiration.org/

> Fantastic resource if you want to delve into yin yoga and TCM further. Jo Phee is a clear and inspiring teacher who fuses holistic oriental medicine with functional anatomy and movement.

https://yinyoga.com/

> A valuable website for all things yin yoga, provided by Bernie Clark. You can find detailed descriptions and videos of all yin yoga asanas here.

Recommended Reading (along with My Bibliography)

Baird, Julia. *Phosphorescence: On Awe, Wonder and Things That Sustain You When the World Goes Dark*. Sydney, Australia: Harper Collins Publishers, 2020.

Bradley, K, and N Ritar. *Milkwood: Real Skills for Down-to-Earth Living*. Sydney: Murdoch Books, 2018.

Elliot-Howery, Alex, and Jaimee Edwards. *Use It All: The Cornersmith Guide to a More Sustainable Kitchen*. Sydney: Murdoch Books, 2021.

Kornfield, Jack. *A Path with Heart: A Guide through the Perils and Promises of a Spiritual Life*. New York & Toronto: Bantam Books, 1993.

Miles, Jade. *Future-Steading: Live Like Tomorrow Matters*. Sydney, NSW: Murdoch Books, 2021.

Pascoe, Bruce. *Dark Emu*. Broome: Magabala Books, 2014.

Purbrick, Matt, and Lentil. *The Village: Good Food, Gardening and Nourishing Traditions to Feed Your Village*. Sydney: Pan Macmillan, 2018.

Stuart, Alexx. *Low Tox Life: A Handbook for a Healthy You and a Happy Planet*. Sydney: Murdoch Books, 2018.

Stuart, Alexx. *Low Tox Food: How to Shop, Cook, Swap, Save and Eat for a Happy Planet*. Sydney: Murdoch Books, 2021.

Whitton, Jo, and Comerford, Elyse. *Simple, Healing Food*. Self-published, Quirky Cooking, 2021.

Whitton, Jo, and Kassab, Fouad. *Life-Changing Food*. Self-published, 2017.

Endnotes

Chapter 1 Endnotes

1 Jennifer Isaacs, ed., *Australian Dreaming: 40,000 Year of Aboriginal History* (Australia: New Holland Publishers, 2005), 99.

2 Tyson Yunkaporta, *Sand Talk: How Indigenous Thinking Can Save the World* (The Text Publishing Company, 2019), 275. Tyson kindly gave permission for me to quote him in this book.

3 Thich Nhat Hanh, *Teachings on Love* (Parallax Press), 1997.

4 Lao Tzu is also known as Laozi and/or Lao-Tze.

5 Daniel Reid, *The Tao of Health, Sex, and Longevity: A Modern, Practical Approach to the Ancient Way* (London: Simon and Schuster, 1989), 3.

6 Reid, *The Tao of Health, Sex, and Longevity.*

7 Jo Phee is one of my revered teachers of yin yoga and TCM. She has kindly permitted me to include her words of wisdom dotted throughout this book.

Chapter 2 Endnotes

1 X. C. Dopico, M. Evangelou, R. C. Ferreira, H. Guo, M. L. Pelalski, D. J. Smyth, N. Cooper, O. S. Burren, A. J. Fulford, B. J. Hennig, A. M. Prentice, A-G Ziegler, E Bonifaco, C. Wallace, J. A. Todd. "Widespread Seasonal Gene Expression Reveals Annul Differences in Human Immunity and Physiology," *Nature Communications* (May 2015).

2 Museums Victoria, "Seven Seasons of the Kulin Peoples," https://museumsvictoria.com.au/melbournemuseum/resources/forest-secrets/.

3 Wendell Berry, "The Peace of Wild Things," in *New Collected Poems* (Minneapolis: Graywolf Press, 2012). Copyright © 2012 by Wendell Berry. Reprinted with the permission of The Permissions Company, LLC on behalf of Counterpoint Press, counterpointpress.com., LLC on behalf of Graywolf Press, Minneapolis, Minnesota, graywolfpress.org.

4 Robin Wall Kimmerer, *Braiding Sweetgrass: Indigenous Wisdom, Scientific Knowledge, and the Teachings of Plants* (Penguin UK, 2020), 9.

Chapter 4 Endnotes

1 Lao Tzu is a past poet and philosopher from China who is said to have written the *Tao Te Ching*, a very long and famous poem, approximately 2,500 years ago.

2 G. K. Chesterton, "Chapter 1," in *Tremendous Trifles*, first published by Methuen, 1909.

3 Kristin D. Neff, "The Development and Validation of a Scale to Measure Self-Compassion," *Self and Identity* 2, no. 3: 223–50, DOI: 10.1080/15298860309027.

4 Jo Phee is one of my revered teachers of yin yoga and TCM. She has kindly permitted me to include her words of wisdom dotted throughout this book.

5 His Holiness the Dalai Lama, Archbishop Desmond Tutu, and Douglas Abrams, *The Book of Joy: Lasting Happiness in a Changing World* (UK: Penguin Random House, 2016).

Chapter 5 Endnotes

1 N. Farb, J. Daubenmier, C. J. Price, T. Gard, C. Kerr, B. D. Dunn, A. C. Klein, M. P. Paulus, and W. E. Mehling. "Interoception, Contemplative Practice, and Health," *Front Psychology* 9, no. 6 (June 2015): 763. Doi: 10.3389/fpsyg.2015.00763. PMID: 26106345; PMCID: PMC4460802.

2 Fascia Research Congress information, https://fasciacongress.org/congress/fascia-glossary-of-terms/.

3 Fascia Research Congress.

4 Sarah Powers, *Insight Yoga* (Boulder: Shambala Publications, 2008), 18.

5 Bernie Clark, *The Complete Guide to Yin Yoga: The Philosophy and Practice of Yin Yoga*, 1ˢᵗ ed. (Vancouver, B.C., Canada: Wild Strawberry Productions, 2018), 34.

6 Jo Phee is one of my revered teachers of Yin yoga and TCM. She has kindly permitted me to include her words of wisdom and insight throughout this book.

7 FeetUp Trainers, https://feetup.com.au/ https://feetup.com/.

Chapter 6 Endnotes

1 Roderik J. S. Gerritsen and Guido P. H. Band, "Breath of Life: The Respiratory Vagal Stimulation Model of Contemplative Activity" *Frontiers in Human Neuroscience* (first published online, October 9, 2018). DOI: 10.3389/fnhum.2018.00397.

2 Gerritsen and Band, "Breath of Life."

Chapter 7 Endnotes

1 Bob Sharples, *Meditation: Calming the Mind* (Lothian, 2003). Reprinted with kind permission from Bob Sharples.

2 Kaveri Patel, "A New and Deeper Truth," in *Under the Waves* (2012). Reprinted with kind permission from Kaveri Patel.

3 William Stafford, "The Way It Is," in *Ask Me:100 Essential Poems* (Minneapolis, Minnesota: Graywolf Press, 1977, 2004). Copyright 1977, 2004 by William Stafford and the Estate of William Stafford. Reprinted with the permission of The Permissions Company, LLC on behalf of Graywolf Press, Minneapolis, Minnesota, graywolfpress.org.

4 Ian Gawler and Paul Bedson, *Meditation: An In-Depth Guide* (Australia: Allen & Unwin Publishers, 2010). Reprinted with kind permission from Paul Bedson & Ian Gawler.

Chapter 8 Endnotes

1 Michael Lane, MD, and Vijayshree Yadav MD, MCR, FAAN, in *Textbook of Natural Medicine*, 5ᵗʰ ed. (2020), https://www.sciencedirect.com/book/9780323523424/textbook-of-natural-medicine.

2 Jaana Suvisaari, "Outi Mantere," in *The Innate Immune Response to Noninfectious Stressors* (2016).

3 T. G. Dinan and J. F. Cryan, "The Impact of Gut Microbiota on Brain and Behavior: Implications for Psychiatry, *Current Opinion in Clinical Nutrition and Metabolic Care* 18, no. 6 (November 2015): 552–58.

4 Rumi is a well-known Persian poet from the thirteenth century.

5 Dave Apsrey, *Fast This Way: Burn Fat, Heal Inflammation and Eat Like the High-Performing Human You Were Meant to Be* (Harper Collins Publishers, 2021), 215.

Chapter 9 Endnotes

1 Rumi is a well-known Persian poet from the thirteenth century.

2 Lao Tzu is a past poet and philosopher from China who is said to have written the *Tao Te Ching*, a very long and famous poem, approximately 2,500 years ago.

Chapter 10 Endnotes

1 Paul Pitchford, *Healing with Whole Foods: Asian Traditions and Modern Nutrition*, 3ʳᵈ ed.

2 Albert Camus was a French author, journalist, and philosopher. At age forty-four, he was awarded the 1957 Nobel Prize in literature.

3 Rumi is a well-known Persian poet from the thirteenth century.

Chapter 11 Endnotes

1 Jo Phee is one of my revered teachers of yin yoga and TCM. She has kindly permitted me to include her words of wisdom and insight throughout this book.

2 Kaveri Patel, "Spacious," in *The Voice* (2014). Reprinted with kind permission from Kaveri Patel.

Chapter 12 Endnotes

1 Paul Pitchford, *Healing with Whole Foods: Asian Traditions and Modern Nutrition*, 3rd ed.

2 Michael Leunig is an Australian cartoonist, writer, painter, philosopher, and poet. You can find more of his wonderful works via *The Age* newspaper, *The Sydney Morning Herald*, his books, and his website (http://www.leunig.com.au/).

3 His Holiness the Dalai Lama, Archbishop Desmond Tutu, and Douglas Abrams, *The Book of Joy: Lasting Happiness in a Changing World* (UK: Penguin Random House UK, 2016), 261.

4 Kaveri Patel, "Breathe into Your Heart," in *Awakening* (2021). Reprinted with kind permission from Kaveri Patel.

Chapter 13 Endnotes

1 Mary Oliver, *Swan: Poems and Prose Poems* (Boston: Beacon Press, 2010). Reprinted by permission of the Charlotte Sheedy Literary Agency Inc.

Chapter 14 Endnotes

1 Permission was kindly given to reproduce this information from the Miriam Rose Foundation.

2 Miriam-Rose Ungunmerr (1988). All Rights Reserved. Permission was kindly granted to reproduce part of Miriam-Rose's reflection here by the Miriam Rose Foundation.

3 The recipe for Life-Changing Gluten Free Sough-Dough Crumpets can be found in Matt and Lentil Purbrick's *Grown and Gathered: Traditional Living Made Modern* (Plum, 2016).

Index

I wish you all the best with your practice.
Attune and Bloom.
XX Freya

Lightning Source UK Ltd.
Milton Keynes UK
UKHW052237110722
405692UK00005B/214

9 781982 293826